D1715258

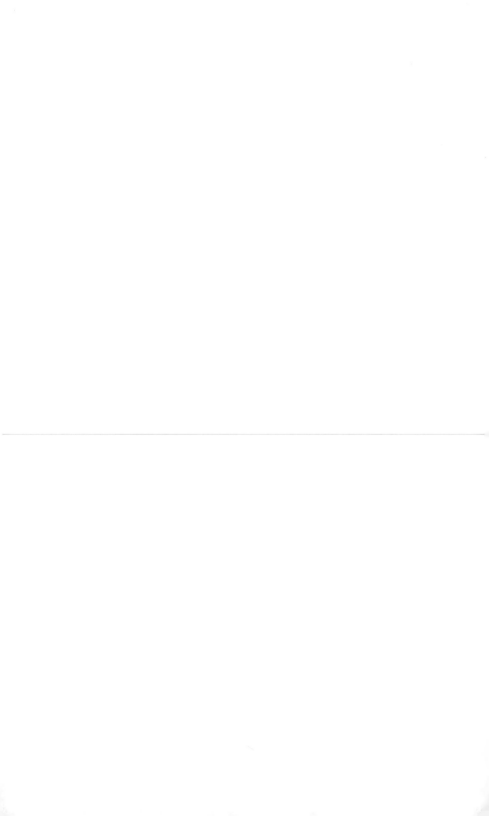

Philosophical and Historical Roots of Occupational Therapy

Philosophical and Historical Roots of Occupational Therapy

Karen Diasio Serrett, PhD, OTR, FAOTA
Editor

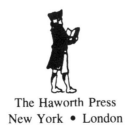

The Haworth Press
New York • London

Philosophical and Historical Roots of Occupational Therapy has also been published as *Occupational Therapy in Mental Health,* Volume 5, Number 3, Fall 1985.

The Haworth Press, Inc., 28 East 22 Street, New York, NY 10010
EUROSPAN/Haworth, 3 Henrietta Street, London WC2E 8LU England

Library of Congress Cataloging in Publication Data
Main entry under title:

Philosophical and historical roots of occupational therapy.

    Has also been published as: Occupational in therapy mental health, v. 5, no. 3, fall 1985.
    Reprinted from various sources.
    Includes bibliographies.
    1. Occupational therapy—History—Addresses, essays, lectures. 2. Mental illness—Treatment—History—Addresses, essays, lectures. 3. Psychobiology—Addresses, essays, lectures. I. Serrett, Karen Diasio. [DNLM: 1. Mental Disorders—therapy—collected works. 2. Mental Health—collected works. 3. Occupational Therapy—history—collected works. W1 0C601N v.5, no.3 / WM 11.1 H6733]
RC487.P48 1985   616.89'165   85-8838
ISBN 0-86656-456-X
ISBN 0-86656-527-2 (soft)

Philosophical and Historical Roots of Occupational Therapy

Occupational Therapy in Mental Health
Volume 5, Number 3

CONTENTS

BETH MOYER, MS, OTR, FAOTA, *Occupational Therapy Consultant, Florida State Hospital, Chattahoochee, FL*

ANNE C. MOSEY, PhD, OTR, *Professor, Department of Occupational Therapy, New York University, New York, NY*

FRANCES OAKLEY, MS, OTR, *Consultant, Occupational Therapy Service, National Institutes of Health, Clinical Center, Bethesda, MD*

SUSAN CLEARY SCHWARTZ, OTR, *Program Coordinator, Inpatient Psychiatry, Pacific Medical Center, San Francisco, CA*

DIANE SHAPIRO, MA, OTR, *Division of Therapeutic Activities, The New York Hospital-Cornell Medical Center, Westchester Division, White Plains, NY*

JANE SLAYMAKER, MA, OTR, FAOTA, *Associate Professor, Occupational Therapy Department, University of Florida, Gainesville, FL*

FRANKLIN STEIN, PhD, OTR, *Director, Occupational Therapy Program, University of Wisconsin, Milwaukee, WI*

MARY SAVAGE STOWELL, MS, OTR, *Consultant, Bainbridge Is., WA*

JOYCE WARD, MS, OTR, *Chair, Department of Research, The Sheppard and Enoch Pratt Hospital, Towson, MD*

GERALD WHITMARSH, PhD, *Director of Research, The Sheppard and Enoch Pratt Hospital, Towson, MD*

Preface

The purpose of this special issue on the history of the profession of occupational therapy, particularly in mental health, is to highlight some key aspects of thinking about occupational therapy's evolution and its initial sense of purpose, in a way that acknowledges, articulates, and brings forth our roots in a rich intellectual tradition that has direct linkages with the emerging Systems Age. Appropriate choices then can be made in the reconciling of critical issues facing the occupational therapy profession that allows it to make its best possible contribution to society over time.

Much of that intellectual tradition, at the inception of occupational therapy as a formal discipline, is unknown to present-day therapists and other professionals. In reprinting papers, articles, chapters, and quotes from that era, it is my hope that we as occupational therapists may find intellectual nurturance and increased *will* toward our basic professional mission, and a deeply satisfying sense of our own early identity and *being* as a professional group that will complement our always-strong desire toward excellence in doing and *function*.

Karen Diasio Serrett, PhD, OTR, FAOTA
Professor
Department of Occupational Therapy
San Jose State University

Acknowledgements

Special thanks to James V. Clark and Charles G. Krone for their enduring contributions to my own thinking as a human being, as an occupational therapist and as an organizational consultant.

Karen Diasio Serrett, PhD, OTR, FAOTA

Philosophical and Historical Roots of Occupational Therapy

Another Look
at Occupational Therapy's History:
Paradigm or Pair-of-Hands?

Karen Diasio Serrett

THE GROWING INTERNAL DEBATE

Over the past two decades, leaders in occupational therapy have been focused on developing a more adequate theory base and grounding occupational therapy in a philosophy that clarifies for us what is of enduring value. Practitioners, however, have sought improvements in the clinical skills needed in their settings, where conditions are shifting so rapidly as to be breathtaking. These are, in many ways, dissimilar solutions to emergent trends and shifts that are awesome in scope. Above all, the rate of change itself is accelerating, and the resultant complexity is what we are all struggling to manage, albeit in differing ways (Beer, 1975).

One fundamental change that is occurring is in the way we view the world and its events. Called paradigm shifts by Thomas Kuhn, they have not only been described for occupational therapy (Diasio, 1981, Kielhofner & Burke, 1977, Guilfoyle, 1984) but also for science in general (Ackoff, 1982, Capra, 1981, Fergusen, 1980). Russell Ackoff has characterized this shift as the greatest major change in our thinking since the Renaissance. The Renaissance, he claims, ushered in the Machine Age which produced the Industrial Revolution. The current intellectual revolution is bringing in a new era he calls the Systems Age which is producing the Post-Industrial Revolution. Changes between these ages, he contends, are both giving rise to the crises we face as well as offering hope to deal with them effectively (1977, 1982).

Increasing world complexity, seen in the environmental turbulence all around us, requires new capabilities, especially in think-

Karen Diasio Serrett, PhD, OTR, FAOTA, is Professor, Occupational Therapy Department, San Jose State University.

1

ing about how to manage. A fundamental reconceptualization of what we are capable of, declares Beer, is required: from Homo Faber (man the maker) to Homo Gubernator (man the regulator). Thus, the answer can no longer simply be in making and doing more, since the technologies that have come from that focus have created problems that are no longer solvable by more of the same. The answer must come from getting the mind to manage the complexity in a new way, using new capabilities of thinking (Beer, 1975).

For organizations, these changing world realities, characterized by increasing environmental turbulence, require fundamental shifts in management tasks (Kanter, 1983). Organizations must now continually compete for scarce resources. The critical shifts in management tasks that Kanter foresees impact all levels of the organization. Top management needs to spend increasing amounts of time dealing with environmental changes going on outside the organization, since there are increasing constraints with which top managers must contend. They must devote much more time in interfacing with external stakeholders: customers, regulatory agencies, funding sources, and the like. At the bottom of the organization, there are increased demands for freedom and autonomy in the worksite; workers expect higher quality of worklife and freedom to apply their skills, participating in decisions affecting their work life. Those in middle management, she states, increasingly need to deal with issues of power, meaning the ability to mobilize resources to get things done. Increasingly, those in middle management will be called to demonstrate the efficacy of their services, and will need to deal with power issues in myriad forms. New organizational forms such as task forces, steering committees, and matrix organizations, call for managers who can handle much responsibility without the traditional authority prerogatives that used to attend them.

Occupational therapists, increasingly in middle and top management positions, can undoubtedly recognize the validity of these shifting managerial tasks. A sea change is occurring in our environments, one that has to do at heart with accountability for results in every arena. We are currently witnessing the transformation of health and human services into businesses. In health care, it has meant the adoption of cost containment measures to slow down exploding costs. At present, accountability is being widely translated into concern for bottom line dollar figures as the primary measure of effectiveness, although that is only one of many that will need to be addressed.

Indeed, since the cutbacks of the last recession, the managerial demands on occupational therapists in mental health have accelerated markedly. Most therapists are both delivering direct services to clients and carrying increasing responsibilities for managerial tasks in the system. Most promotional opportunities are opening for those who do well in the managerial areas and those who can facilitate efficient and effective team accomplishment. Thus, there is real opportunity in these shifting times. Conversely, for those who are ill-prepared for these demands, burnout is the more likely result. The antidote for burnout, then, is an increase in capability in conceiving the opportunities, in a new way of thinking.

Our literature for over a decade is replete with leaders in occupational therapy who are increasingly concerned with our collective ability to manage the dramatic changes occurring in systems around us in the health and human service arenas, bringing us a recurring message. Time and again that essential message is: improve our collective professional capability! Fidler warns that there is a growing rift between the leaders of the profession and the average practitioner:

> There is an uncomfortable distance between our leaders and our common practice. . . . Until we deal with our need for increased professional education, the distance between our leaders and common practice will grow. Achievement of a sense of competence on the part of practitioners will remain an elusive goal. (1981, p. 572)

Thus, leaders are trying to activate new levels of capability as they see the demands growing for adaptability and evolution given increased demands from the public and society for accountability. Practitioners, who want more skills but want ones that can help them in their jobs, resist the emphasis on philosophy and theory. Fox's study shows that new graduates do not place high priority on theory development, and resist learning the theory behind new techniques and methods (Fox, 1981). Yet another study by Allen and Cruickshank (1977) showed that beginning therapists are most bothered by issues related to management of time, and issues related to dealing with other professionals on a mutually respectful basis. Particularly bothersome was "getting other professionals to understand and respect the role of occupational therapy" (p. 562). They concluded that

> Therapists need to identify what functions are indicated and accomplishable within whatever system and arena they find themselves. They then need to present their services from a strong theoretical base within those boundaries. This is not to say that systems cannot be changed. They might be more easily changed from a strong and respected base within the system. (p. 563)

Competence was a third area of bothersome problems, having to do with development of self-confidence and the ability to assert one's professional self as an outgrowth of reliable effective service that is demonstrable and recompensable. It would seem that in a very short time, new therapists are confronted with demands they cannot easily reckon with. Their notions of what they need is at variance with what many of the profession's leaders see is needed for professional viability. Furthermore, the professional association has been slow to move in reconciling these different perceptions. The problems cited in these more recent research studies, interestingly enough, bear a marked resemblance to those of Crampton and Anderegg's study reported in 1961. In that study, psychiatric occupational therapists in Massachusetts state hospitals reported the lack of communication and understanding between occupational therapists and other staff with resultant uncertainty and job stress.

In the meanwhile, though, evidence is being accumulated as to what is the nature of the problems we face as a professional group. In 1976, the Mental Health Task Force identified issues for occupational therapy in mental health as being related to professional uncertainty, and called for theory building, research, and a move to graduate level professional entry. In 1977, the Ad Hoc Committee on Education, looking at the university systems in which occupational therapy curricula must stay viable, also identified the preparation of clinicians at the baccalaureate level as a source of many existing and continuing problems, along with lack of support in the professional association for persons seeking higher positions and qualifications, especially at master and doctoral levels. Rogers and Mann (1980) showed that professional productivity was positively correlated with masters' level education for occupational therapists.

Radowsky (1980) showed that published occupational therapists were more likely to hold graduate degrees. Data from the Commission of Education's Committee to Review Educational Essentials (AOTA, 1981), showed that therapists in both clinical and academic setting stated that the baccalaureate adequately prepared occupational therapists for the clinical role at entry, but not for research, administrative, or consulting roles, which many felt could only be acquired with experience or graduate education. A study of job performance and personality of occupational therapists in Canada (Peacock & O'Shea, 1984) shows occupational therapists studied were high on nurturance, indicating a need to give sympathy and care, and high on desirability, reflecting a need for social approval and support, and low on exhibition, indicating the desire not to attract attention to themselves. The authors cited another study in Canada (Max, 1978) that showed one of the two most significant problems for occupational therapists was a lack of a clearly defined area of competence. They felt the lack of a clear profile might indicate that occupational therapy does not project a clear image to applicants.

At the specially convened "Occupational Therapy: 2001" in 1978, a number of our leaders gathered with our decision-makers in Scottsdale, Arizona to consider future directions for occupational therapy. Themes emerged that primarily aimed at seeing that we were at a crossroad in deciding whether occupational therapy would evolve as a professional or a technical group. Wilma West spoke of our current state of occupational therapy thinking and development, using the analogy of the human system. Activities were the core or trunk of the profession, the bases in biological, social and psychological sciences its legs, and the applications in clinical practice its arms. The brain or mind of the profession, which controls the whole, were in embryonic state (West, 1978).

In 1979, the Editorial Board of *Occupational Therapy in Mental Health,* who are professional leaders in the mental health area of occupational therapy, engaged in an open systems planning approach to the journal and identified in 1979 the issues and trends affecting occupational therapy in mental health. They included (1) demonstrating effectiveness through research, (2) improving practice, deriving from a theory base, (3) understanding, dealing with, making decisions about, and increasing viability regarding outside forces, (4) defining our philosophical base and theoretical body of knowledge, and finally, (5) improving educational processes. When asked the significance of these issues, virtually all respondees indicated these areas are currently inadequate and need improvement. Thus, the initial mission and core process of *Occupational Therapy in Mental Health* was to *expand capability through conceptualization* (Diasio, 1980).

One of the clearest issues to emerge has to do with the development of the thinking necessary to manage complexity and meet new demands. Many leaders in occupational therapy thus acknowledge the factors Kanter describes: increasing turbulence in society calls for new and different levels of expertise and skill in top and middle management. These thinking capabilities, which underly our ability to manage ourselves effectively, will be used in demonstrating to stakeholders in health and human services (including regulatory bodies, third party payers, and consumers) that occupational therapy gives services worthy of support from society. Many of the membership seem reluctant to share this same sense of urgency in rising to meet these escalating demands, or do not see that such demands will require shifts in professional competencies or requirements, or the reallocation of professional association resources and focus. Other leaders who are reluctant to endorse solutions that have been proposed thus far, seem to want more thorough thinking about the potential impacts of such solutions before acting. One could indeed see the issues as primarily posing a crisis for the leadership who are trying to activate new capabilities in the profession. What will they do if the decisions that are made (even if by not making them) do not support their visions of where we need to go? Can we afford to lose those visions or those leaders?

LEARNING FROM HISTORY

Since this great internal debate shows no signs of abating, what would help to move us forward? It is my premise that another look at the history of thought and its impact on the transformations in occupational therapy has yet more to inform us about our future professional choices. What intellectual heritage exists upon which we can systematically build in bringing about a decisive paradigm shift in occupational therapy? Can lessons emerge from another look at our history that might reconcile the issues in the great internal debate, and that can assist us in freeing our energies to make choices consistent with both our dramatic growth in recent decades and the new levels of complexity with which we must deal? That is both the purpose of this paper and of this special issue.

To do so, we will travel some roads explored and some relatively unexplored in our ongoing search for the essence of our identity and meaning. We will in particular look at the patterns of thought which both expanded and concentrated our practice. My own personal journey in the search for our roots began nearly twenty years ago when Bob Bing told me to look up Meyer's "Philosophy of Occupation Therapy," at a time it was only available in archives. The quality of thinking in that paper filled me with wonder. A question emerged for me which I have never forgotten: what on earth happened in the intervening years that seemed to take us away from that kind of thinking? Since then, a search for our roots has taught me much about what I find most exciting and inspiring in this profession, casting a new light on the issues we need to reappraise. The journey starts with some premises about the components necessary to sustain and evolve toward a better future. It searches for the dominant modes of thought that coevolved with the appearance of occupational therapy. It will look at the assumptions of both the Machine Age and the Systems Age, as described by Ackoff, and how they affected the practice of occupational therapy (even before it assumed that name) from moral treatment to present times. We will examine closely the philosophical roots of occupational therapy arising from the thinking of the functionalist school of psychology and the pragmatist school of philosophy, and examine a division of labor at the inception of occupational therapy that has had long-lasting effects on present-day practice. Finally, in reflecting on what can be learned from this journey through our history of thought, it is my hope that some redefined issues will emerge, from which we might draw reconciling principles for the road ahead.

PREMISES IN THINKING ABOUT ORGANIZATIONS

It will first be necessary to state some premises underlying the approach used in this journey through history. It rests on looking at three components to experience that are necessary to sustain an evolutionary path forward, a path where continual improvement and upgrading can emerge. These components are called function, being, and will (Bennett, 1968, 1978).

Function relates to how things work, the doing of things. It is related to that subsystem or component of a living system that Bennett has called the *moving center* (similar to Kielhofner & Burke's performance subsystem).

Being relates to inner togetherness and internal ordering, our centeredness. Being requires the appropriate availability or concentration of the right quality of energy to be released in a given situation (we are always, as living systems, transforming energy). Being relates to the quality of energy brought to bear; it is how we transform ourselves and manage ourselves in the face of sudden change. Being is related, in Bennett's terms, to the *emotional center* (which in Kielhofner & Burke's formulation, there is a partially equivalent counterpart in the description of habituation, which is only one quality of energy).

Will is seen through function—it activates us and shows in our purposes, intentions, and commitments. Many times, in individuals and organizations, will is fragmented into many small pieces because there is no common uniting purpose and vision that commands our actions. Unity of will is experienced rarely, and most often when we can elevate our energy above our habitual patterns of thinking, feeling, and doing. Will is strongly connected, overall, with the *intellectual center* (similar to the volitional subsystem); it is what we choose to put in our minds that determines our will, not solely what the environment puts out in front of us. We still must make a choice about what we will be activated by in the environment.

Most people and organizations have differences in which of these components they are more developed, and which is their "flat side." All need to be in balance to sustain evolutionary growth forward (Krone, 1983). It is through these premises that this paper will explore our history.

THE MORAL TREATMENT ERA

A spirit of optimism characterized the early nineteenth century in America. It was an era of populist sentiment, in a predominantly agrarian-based economy, with small-community living as its dominant lifestyle, and the young country expanding. This spirit of optimism extended toward those with emotional disorders. In small facilities, doctors and patients from similar backgrounds shared common values and participated together in daily living regimens. Former patients were integrated back into a lifestyle and environment that could use their contributions. The birth of moral treatment, according to Bing (1981), was one result of the Age of Enlightenment. Bockoven describes America in the 1830s and 1840s, which was

> rapidly developing a new liberal philosophy of the individual. Leading American thinkers of the period turned to nature in search of truth. Societies were formed for the abolition of slavery. Experiments were made in communal living. A spirit of freedom and self-expression were in the air. New England Puritanism was growing milder. The jealous God of Cotton Mather was becoming the loving God of William Channing, and a new intellectual independence was coming to the fore. Emerson encouraged the individual to self-reliance. . . . Historically, in the United States, this period has been referred to by Fisher as "The Rise of the Common Man, 1820-1850."

Bockoven also cites the beliefs of the era: that stress could result from disappointment. Such stresses were called moral causes, and their treatment was, of course, moral treatment. This meant that

> the patient was made comfortable, his interest aroused, his friendship invited, and discussion of his troubles encouraged. His time was managed and filled with purposeful activity. (p. 172)

American thought was also influenced by thinking in Europe. The work of Pinel of France, during the French Revolution, became known in this country, as was that of Tuke of England. American psychiatry was influenced by the psychobiological approach taken in Germany (Bockoven, 1956, p. 174), especially by the work of Von Feuchtersleben.

In scope, moral treatment was very broad and also very successful. Let us look at how it was described by Butler, a leader of moral treatment, in 1843:

> [Moral treatment] consists of the wholesome discipline of the well-regulated household, regular hours for food and for sleep, manual employment, reading, lectures, and other intellectual exercises and entertainments, and various recreations and amusements, both within and without. . . . The great object of this treatment is to procure a healthful exercise of the body, to abstract the mind from its delusions, to win back the

patient to the regular and useful habits and practices of his former life. (quoted in Harms, 1964)

One cannot help but be awed by the extent of the programs described in the moral treatment era, as well as by their success. Occupation was a primary, rather than an ancillary, mode of treatment, and was practiced by people who held strongly to an optimistic perspective of the person and of society's ability to meet people's needs.

THE INDUSTRIAL REVOLUTION
AND THE MACHINE AGE

Several important trends and influences in the latter half of the nineteenth century contributed to the eclipse of moral treatment. The first Industrial Revolution radically altered the relationship between people and their environments. Urbanization hastened; mechanization of work caused people to be treated as machines and fitted as parts into greater wholes defined primarily by technology and business needs. The country was shaken to its foundations by the Civil War and its aftermath, in a melange of conflicting values and economics. Masses of immigrants, most poverty-stricken, crowded into the cities to find work in the factories. Their values and lifestyles differed from those of the New Englanders, creating gaps in mental health care providers' outlooks that were not to be bridged. Hospitals became crowded with "foreign insane paupers" (Bockoven, 1963). The evolutionary theories of Darwin were used by Sumners to create a social darwinism which held that survival of the fittest did not dictate concern for the immigrant insane.

MENTALITY IN THE MACHINE AGE

Ackoff describes three characteristics of Machine Age thinking that can be helpful in assessing events of this era: reductionism, analysis, and mechanism (Ackoff, 1974). The Machine Age view of the world was that everything is made up of parts. In many of the scientific inquiries of that time, scholars and scientists were studying the ultimate limits of taking things apart, called *reductionism*. Secondly, the *mode* of thinking used in the Machine Age was *analysis,* so that if one wants to solve a problem, one proceeds by taking it apart. Problems are solved by making aggregates of solutions into a total solution. Thirdly, *mechanism* is based on relating all phenomena into cause-and-effect chains. Ackoff describes the peculiar consequences of this idea: if one event is a necessary and sufficient cause of another event, then nothing else is necessary to explain it; the explanation is complete. Therefore, Ackoff maintains, the concept of environment was irrelevant in classical science.

It is fascinating to review the demise of moral treatment in this light. Bockoven observed that

> The observation by pathologists of microscopic lesions in the central nervous system of patients who had been mentally ill made a profound impression on many psychiatrists. Mental illness, they concluded, could not be expected to become understandable through study of the patient's behavior. The behavior of the mentally ill could no longer be endowed with meaning having to do with the environment when it was looked upon as a result of mechanical defect in the central control station of the body. . . . Psychiatry . . . accepted the then-current notion of science that all phenomena were reducible to simple material units. Mental illness was looked upon simply as the result of damaged brain material . . . and the seemingly necessary conclusion that mental illness was incurable. . . . Scientific psychiatry thus eliminated moral treatment as a definitive therapy and retained it in diluted form as a diversionary adjunct to medical treatment which consisted almost entirely of rest and diet. (p. 189)

This mode of science was not limited to psychiatry. It was, rather, the dominant mode of thinking in the structural school of psychology, and in other sciences as well.

NEW THINKING AT THE TURN OF THE CENTURY

The time preceding occupational therapy's formal birth was in many ways an unusual one in United States history. The general atmosphere of the Progressive Era was once again that of optimism and humanitarianism, which repudiated the social darwinism and rugged individualism of the previous era (Musto, 1975). Sicherman characterized that era as one of social and political reform:

A new intellectual outlook made physicians and laymen less willing to tolerate disease, poverty, and other evils long considered inevitable. The idea that humans could control their environment, instead of passively submitting to it, was of central importance to men and women of this generation. It provided a rationale for such diverse reforms as the elimination of large trusts, establishment of school hygiene programs, well baby clinics and public playgrounds, and legislated public standards of health and welfare. Physicians supported many of these ventures and cooperated with laymen in the new voluntary health organizations that sprang up after 1904 to eliminate TB, infant mortality, mental illness, cancer and venereal disease. Optimism ran so high that some physicians proclaimed disease "largely a removable evil." Americans hoped not just to cure or prevent illness, but to enhance the quality of life itself. (1975, p. 21)

Three unique streams from psychiatry, psychology and social science, and philosophy which emerged in the Progressive Era were the ground of thinking from which occupational therapy drew its life and initial vision. The unity in their collective vision, which spread through American society, is both inspiring and even astounding; these were leaders who truly made a difference in people's lives. Interestingly, the major proponents of these streams were often considered leading thinkers in more than one discipline, which seems uniquely appropriate to their holistic message. James and Dewey, for example, are known as both psychologists and philosophers. Scholars tend to describe their contribution as wide-ranging and hard to classify; their methods were eclectic.

The functionalist school in psychology and social science, which included John Dewey, George Herbert Mead, Charles Peirce, Branislaw Malinowski, and William James, represented a revolt against the preceding structural school of thought, where the focus was on attempts to identify elements of consciousness (psychology) or physical characteristics (anthropology), with laboratory experimentation as the prescribed methodology.

Structuralism aligned with the predominant scientific modes which Ackoff described: reductionism, analysis, cause-and-effect determinism. The functionalists challenged this focus and determined to ask very different questions in psychology related to people as biological units (including an emphasis on both consciousness and activity) using processes of their minds to function and adapt in their environments. William James' brilliant works took issue with notions of the structuralists that consciousness could be reduced to its elements studied separately from life. James' famous paper on habit, so influential in the establishment of Slagle's habit-training programs in occupational therapy, appears elsewhere in this volume (James, 1892). Consciousness, he asserted, served the purpose of adapting humans to their environments through a distinction between conscious choice and habit.

Peirce's and Dewey's social philosophy of pragmatism focused on the needs for humans to use their minds and hands in adapting to life circumstances, with Dewey finally focusing much of his efforts in education. Dewey, in his famous paper "The Reflex Arc in Psychology," attacked the elementalism and reductionism of the reflex arc with its distinction between stimulus and response (Dewey, 1896). He argued that behavior cannot be reduced to these elements any more than consciousness can be analyzed by its elementary components (Schultz, 1960). More important is that behavior be studied in its significance to the organism adapting to its environment, and that this be the primary task of psychology. Dewey is known not only as a psychologist, but as a philosopher and educator. The influence of the functional-pragmatic school can be readily seen in Burnham's educational text, *The Normal Mind* (1924):

> In the individual, integration and the power of adjustment may be developed, physically, by coordinated activity, and mentally, in the doing of purposeful tasks. By the doing of tasks, mental attitudes are developed, and they, together with inherited tendencies, determine behavior. (p. 677)

Not coincidentally, Burnham quotes extensively from Meyer's "Philosophy of Occupation Therapy" in describing and advocating proper mental hygiene for teachers of school children (pp. 617-619).

Dewey's notions of evolution had much more benign implications than those of Sumner's social darwinism. His philosophy advocated social change and progress through consciousness bringing about appropriate activity enabling survival and progress. Dewey, James, and Meyer stressed thinking processes and consciousness used for activities in adapting to environmental demands. Schultz describes their view:

A function is a total coordination of an organism toward achieving an end—survival. Functional psychology is thus the study of the organism "in use". . . . [Dewey] considered man's psychological processes, such as thinking and learning, to be of paramount importance in his adjustments to life. Thinking, he said, was a tool used by man to meet the exigencies of life: man thinks in order to live. (p. 126)

Malinöwski viewed society as a body of institutions related to the current adaptive needs of humans:

the functional view of culture set down the principle that in every type of civilisation, every custom, material object, idea and belief fulfills some vital function, has some task to accomplish, represents an indispensible part within a working whole. (Kardiner & Preble, 1961, p. 151)

Their methods of scientific inquiry were wide-ranging but focused on naturalistic rather than laboratory study. In anthropology in particular, Malinowski insisted on participant observation and qualitative as well as quantitative studies. In any case, the functionalists reconceptualized psychology, regarding natural events in the natural world as worthy of study. One of their greatest contributions was to redefine what psychologists would ask as their basic questions for scientific inquiry. Theirs was a focus on the commonsense, as was Meyer's in psychiatry. Their very acceptance and success in this redefinition eventually contributed to their fading from view in the middle decades of the twentieth century. The collaborative and shared nature of their beliefs and values and their wide-ranging impact on science, government, philosophy, and the arts (Kardiner & Preble, 1961) have since been shrouded from view by the tendency of each discipline to report its history separate from the others.

Most occupational therapists are familiar with Adolf Meyer's contribution to the theoretical foundations of the profession in his seminal paper, "Philosophy of Occupation Therapy." Meyer was both part of a larger movement and himself created streams within it, such as the mental hygiene movement and "commonsense psychiatry." The larger movement of which Meyer was part was the functional-pragmatist one of psychology and philosophy. Meyer had close friendships with James, Dewey, Peirce, who were some of its leading thinkers, and shared a common perspective with them (Lidz, 1966).

Meyer, who began in medicine as a neuropathologist, led the attack against strict elementalism in psychiatry:

> The human organism can never exist without its setting in the world. All we are and do is of the world and in the world. The great mistake of an overambitious science has been the desire to study man altogether as a mere sum of parts, if possible of atoms, or now of electrons, and as a machine, detached, by itself, because at least some points in the simpler sciences could be studied to the best advantage with this method of the so-called elementalist. It was a long time before willingness to see the large group of facts, in their broad relations as well as in their inner structure, finally gave us the concept and vision of integration which now fits man as a live unit and transformer of energy into the world of fact and makes him frankly a consciously integrated psychobiological individual and member of a social group. (Lief, 1921)

According to Bockoven, Meyer kindled a spirit of research that awakened American psychiatry out of its hopeless stagnation. He called the new scientific discipline he evolved *psychobiology.* Its elaboration by Muncie (1939) in a text on psychiatry appears elsewhere in this volume.

ANTICIPATING THE SYSTEMS ERA

The importance of Meyer's concepts and contributions, despite American psychiatry's acknowledgement of him, has probably not yet been adequately estimated. His contributions are best acknowledged in the growing light of a newly emerging paradigm, aptly described by Ackoff as the thinking of the new Systems Age, which transcends the earlier Machine Age thinking.

Ackoff states that a series of conceptual breakthroughs of monumental importance have been occurring during this century. He traces this series of events by identifying steps in the evolution of a new form of thinking about events, aided by technological breakthroughs that were significant departures from the early ones of the Industrial Revolution which transformed and replaced modes of physical work done by humans. Suzanne Langer's *Philosophy in a New Key* captured what was going on in science in the early mid-twentieth century by stating that science was moving from atom to *symbol*—something that had no matter. Morris maintained that the fundamental change in science was not symbol alone, but *language*. Shannon stated that it was not language but something larger, of which language was part—namely, *communication*. Weiner, the cybernetician, writing at the same time as Shannon in the 1940s, stated that the new organizing concept was *control*. Finally, von Beralanffy, a biologist, identified that the new organizing concept was *system* (Ackoff, 1974, 1981).

In each of these progressive ideas, *the thinking was going upward toward larger and indivisible wholes,* where the performance of that whole is affected by all its parts or subsystems. This contrasts with the Machine Age thinking *which searched for indivisible parts.* Advances in technology mirrored these analogies; the telephone, telegraph, computer, and hologram did not transform matter nor do physical work. Rather, these technologies generate symbols and information, and even manipulate them. These technologies paved the way for growing acceptance and understanding of the central ideas of the Systems Age.

This emphasis on wholes as contrasted with parts, gave rise to a different kind of thinking. The organizing principles of the emerging Systems Age are expansionism, synthesis, and purposefulness/nondeterministic cause and effect. Thus, in *expansionism,* systems scientifically explores the special properties of wholes and wholeness and their relationships. Secondly, *synthesis* is a mode of thinking looking at a whole not to take it apart, but to see it as part of a still larger whole, the parts in relationship to each other, and as a fundamentally different point of departure for scientific inquiry (Blauberg et al., 1977). The performance of the whole is not the addition of the performance of its parts, but is a consequence of the *relationship* between performance of its parts. Thirdly, in contrast to linear cause-and-effect chains, the environment is seen as central rather than peripheral to what was being studied. Weiner, in showing the purposefulness of cybernetic machines, showed a new way of thinking in which concepts of *purpose* and choice could be dealt with scientifically. One could not understand complex creations without considering the purposes for which they were to be used by the larger system of which they are part. Purpose was related to larger wholes, or environments. Thus, the essential properties of a system taken as a whole derive from the interaction of its parts, not their actions taken separately. Therefore, *when a system is taken apart it loses its essential properties.* Because of this—and this is the critical point—*a system is a whole that cannot be understood by analysis.* (Ackoff, 1981, p. 16)

We can now re-examine Meyer's psychobiological concepts, and beyond that, the new perspective cast on occupational therapy as a professional discipline. Psychobiology rejected dualism, the separation of body and mind as independent substances, claiming that dualism led to mechanistic philosophy. Muncie articulated Meyer's psychobiology in a 1939 medical textbook:

> Man emerges as a special and a higher biological product, including within him all the data of physics and chemistry and zoology, but distinguished by the greater development of delayed reflexes as adaptive reactions, by the vast development and use of symbols, especially those of language, and by the hanging together of all these sensory, motor, and associative performances in a special manner called "conscious." In such a system the old contrast of mental and physical with its prejudicial barriers and insolubilia is replaced by consideration of degrees or levels of integration: Are the facts understood as nonmental, that is, as the qualities and activities of essentially detachable parts, organs, or systems (as treated in anatomy and physiology), or are they only intelligible in terms of mentally integrated performances—of a sort indissolubly a function, overt or implicit, of the total organism and having *meaning* as adaptive responses in a total situation?
>
> Psychobiology then is the study of those functions distinctively human, the things man is best known for, the mentally integrated performances. (1939, pp. 23-24)

Meyer, certainly the major conceptual contributor to occupational therapy's intellectual heritage, clearly anticipated the systems thinking which Ackoff describes, including expansionism, synthesis, and purposefulness. His paper "Philosophy of Occupation Therapy" demonstrates the orderly flow of thinking from those premises into the profession of occupational therapy:

The most important factor in the progress lay undoubtedly in the newer conceptions of mental problems as problems of living, and not merely diseases of a structural and toxic nature on the one hand or of a final lasting constitutional disorder on the other. . . . *Performance* is its own judge and regulator and therefore the most dependable and influential part of our life. Our body is not merely so many pounds of flesh and bone figuring as a machine, with an abstract mind or soul added to it. It is throughout a live organism pulsating with its rhythm of rest and activity, beating time . . . in ever so many ways, most readily intelligible and in the full bloom of its nature when it feels itself as one of those great self-guiding *energy transformers* which constitute the real world of living beings. Our conception of man is that of an organism that maintains and balances itself in the world of reality and actuality by being in active life and active use, i.e., using and living and acting its *time* in harmony with its own nature and the nature about it. It is the *use* that we make of ourselves that gives the ultimate stamp to our every organ. (1922)

Meyer's approach was amazingly holistic and environmentally oriented. Very clearly, Meyer and other functionalist leaders such as Mead, Dewey, James, and others, were decades ahead of their times; they anticipated systems thinking by nearly half a century. The approaches in philosophy, education, and other social sciences that took place in the era of occupational therapy's formal birth were truly remarkable for the aligned thinking between leaders in various professions and the political climate of the time. With such a strong foundation, no wonder that occupational therapy had a beginning mandated by society, by   ysicians, and by hospitals! A bibliography of the time fr   95 to 1925 cited literally hundreds of papers and some '   .itten on the subject of occupation for healing, in a v   . nealth journals (Hospital Library and Service Bure   _).

      , the context for Adolf Meyer's "Philosophy of Occupation rapy" was broader and intellectually richer than most occupational therapists initially realized. The initial focus on purposeful (i.e., directed by the mind) activity and mind-body unity is quite clearly a legacy from the intellectual heritage of our early founders and thinkers, especially as promoted within occupational therapy by Meyer and Slagle.

THE LOSS OF OCCUPATIONAL THERAPY'S
INTELLECTUAL HERITAGE

As occupational therapy moved into new decades, this intellectual heritage virtually vanished from our awareness. *Why?* And what have been the costs of such a profound loss of our intellectual roots? Earlier, the necessity of three aspects of experience to sustain an evolutionary path were mentioned: function, being, and will. It seems clear that they were in evidence during this remarkable period at the turn of the century and shortly thereafter, and at the inception of occupational therapy as a formal discipline. There was a rare unity of will and purpose stretching across many disciplines, and high energy for advancing and bettering humankind. Occupational therapy was very much an integral expression of that era, much as it was implicitly in the earlier era of moral treatment. It is highly likely that many of the early occupational therapists, educated at the better Eastern universities before they took short courses in occupational therapy, shared knowledge of this school of thought. But it did not go forward from there.

An implicit decision was made at the time of occupational therapy's birth that stressed *function* at the expense of *will.* The intellectual nourishment of the founding vision cannot be found in the short training courses or early curricula of occupational therapy. Emphasis was placed on the *doing,* and the field attracted people who liked the *doing.* In courses of a few short months' duration, how could it be otherwise? The spirit of the times supplied the will and the being; it was simply not anticipated that these would be lost over time without further intellectual articulation and enrichment by occupational therapists themselves.

Furthermore, the division of labor between physicians and occupational therapists followed traditional patterns regarding men and women. From its inception, occupational therapists were women, who were to act under the guidance of the physicians, predominantly men. Indeed, it was implicit in Dunton's early book, *Prescribing Occupational Therapy* (1928). Dunton's book was written to educate other physicians in the use of occupational therapy, thus compensating for the lack of exposure of physicians to occupational therapy in medical school. Dunton acknowledged the lack of a scientific base for its efficacy, but proceeded on empirical evidence. In involving physicians as stakeholders, he described occupational therapists as technical assistants who would carry out the physicians' principles in administering practical skills which physicians lacked. Thus, the purpose of his book was to supply the beliefs, philosophies, and principles of occupational therapy for the physician's direction of its design and implementation, which would be done by occupational therapists (Dunton, 1928, p. 11). Woodside, reviewing the history of this period, stated

> The early journals illustrate clearly how tenaciously the doctors clung to the necessity of a medical prescription and/or referral to occupational therapy for their services. Physicians praised the therapist's heart while questioning her knowledge and skills. (1971, p. 229)

Thus, the doing, or function, as well as the being, belonged to the women (occupational therapists), and the conceptualizing about the doing, as well as its intellectual control, belonged to the men (physicians). Thus, early occupational therapy had a split between its practice and its conceptualization, between its function and its will, which decades later brought it into a massive identity crisis as occupational therapists sensed their incompleteness as they strived to move toward full professionalism—the consequences of which still dominate most of our profession's current concerns. The conceptualizations and intellectual foundations, which build will, were outside the boundaries of the profession. In the era of intense shared values when occupational therapy was born, this was not perceived to be a critical factor for the profession's eventual evolution.

The spirit of optimism and reform of the Progressive Era, however, did not survive the Depression; hence the initial unity of purpose, or will, that initially supplied the common vision in occupational therapy, faded slowly from view. In the occupational therapy literature, emphasis continued on function—the acquisition of techniques and the description of programs. In mental health, Meyerian psychobiology was eclipsed by Freudian psychoanalysis, which regarded the Meyerian approach as naive and oversimplified, although it is doubtful they fully understood its basic assumptions. Meyer, on the other hand, was pragmatic enough to accept certain aspects of psychoanalysis, but was specifically critical of Freud's reductionistic emphasis as "too largely an emphasis on a portion of the situation" (Lief, 1948, p. 229). Meyer's criticism of psychoanalysis was clearly aimed at its reductionistic mindset; he warned against too complete a satisfaction . . . in their ultimate, perhaps too exclusive and ready surrender to what . . . I consider as too mechanized and overspecialized and too exclusive a "psychopathology of the unconscious." (Lief, p. 35)

A fascinating example of an account of this transition in a private hospital, from a psychoanalytic perspective, was found in an account of the Austin Riggs Foundation during this time period. Riggs, who clearly held the orientation of psychobiology, met the psychoanalytic tradition with resistance and antagonism, yet it came to prevail in the institution. Riggs adhered to a program of education, insight through the life story, and rehabilitation through a program of exercise, balanced work, play and rest. Finally, a great deal of attention was given to planning the future environment of the patient. As the report indicates,

This problem [of planning the future environment of the patient] was frequently overlooked during those early days of psychoanalysis when the emphasis had shifted to an exclusive effort to understand the role of unconscious forces in the total dynamics of the neurotic process. (p. 56)

The contrast between the psychoanalytic versus the psychobiological is found in this account of a Riggs study done in 1940:

In the 1940 study, an effort was made to characterize the neurotic process in ways which would not be used today. For example, it is spoken of as "a manifestation of a failure to adapt." This places the cart squarely before the horse, since it is the failure to adapt which is the manifestation of the neurotic process. In other contexts, the failure to adapt is attributed to "distorted values," "impractical ideas," "faulty attitudes, habits and ways." This again overlooks the fact that all such traits as values, ideas, attitudes, and habits are themselves manifestations of the neurotic process, rather than its cause. (Kubie, 1960, p. 57)

The account of the history of the hospital documents the early psychobiological approach, called a "benevolent but paternalistic philosophy" run by principles of re-education—obviously not even recognized as influenced by Meyer's psychobiology. The Riggs Center abandoned the policy of re-education because such a program did not take into account sufficiently the fact that internal conflicts in the patient could defeat such hopes, that even when seemingly successful during a patient's stay at Riggs, it was not likely to survive long after he left, and that consequently such a program would be less appropriate for the young patient who had not yet achieved anything and who was in rebellion than for the older patient who had already accomplished something with his life. (p. 84)

In the void that was left in the late 1940s and 1950s at that hospital, the patients existed "in what could only euphemistically be called a laissez-faire era. It should more accurately be labeled 'near chaos'— at least at times" (p. 85). The discontent of nurses, activity leaders, and other support staff were only gradually acknowledged—they were labeled as being uncertain of their roles—before the medical staff acknowledged the "relative chaos." This apparently later led to the reinstitution of activity programs and a therapeutic community model. It was obvious that the authors had no knowledge of the premises or the thinking behind the psychobiological approach, and were convinced of the superiority of the psychoanalytic approach.

Undoubtedly, the general acceptance of the psychobiological principles of Meyer faded as its theory base was no longer acknowledged or developed. It is a compelling example of how ideology, in the name of advancement, can limit what were obviously effective programs. The example given in this hospital was quite parallel to my own experience of the limiting psychoanalytic influence of that period in a number of hospitals, that were inimicable to the basic purposes of occupational therapy. Their theory base, rooted in the analytic determinism of Freud, had little space to acknowledge occupational therapy's contributions, which originated in a different kind of thinking. Occupational therapists of that time were at a loss to articulate or substantiate the theoretical roots of their practice (Crampton & Anderegg, 1961). That period bears a remarkable similarity to the kind of thinking that led to the demise of moral treatment; its emphasis was squarely in the realm of the thinking of the Machine Age—reductionism, mechanism, and analysis.

Occupational therapy, which had concentrated its efforts to upgrade itself in the area of function only, was particularly vulnerable to these ideological shifts. The education and literature of occupational therapy had not exposed therapists to or grounded them in that theory base. The profession had not provided for its own intellectual nourishment in planning for its future. In any case, women were accustomed to receiving direction and a *raison d'etre* from the medical men. When medicine became engulfed in an overwhelmingly reductionistic thinking mode, energy in the occupational therapy field became dispersed, its state of being and identity in question. The initial alignment with physicians such as Meyer had evaporated, and we were alone to chart our destiny, although under the guidance of the American Medical Association. Our interactions with other professions gave evidence of our uncertainty and dispersion; multiple similar disciplines were formed with overlaps which continue to haunt us.

In the meanwhile, though, the paradigm shift that had begun so strongly in the Progressive Era in the social sciences, continued to evolve in the biological and physical sciences, where it gained strength. Particularly notable are the discoveries and developments in quantum physics which have challenged and shaken the Neutonian-Cartesian world view of the Machine Age and have enriched our understanding of wholeness and systems (Ackoff, 1981, Beer, 1975, Capra, 1982, Fergusen, 1980, Bohm, 1980). Thus the evolution into the Systems Age, as described earlier in this paper by Ackoff, is now well underway in a number of scientific and professional disciplines.

The growing discovery and reclaiming of our intellectual heritage has been an exhilarating experience for many occupational therapists who began to hunger for a much deeper understanding and commitment to their profession. Seeing that their contributions really mattered to patients' recovery and/or more successful resumption of community living, increasing numbers of occupational therapists returned to graduate school from the 1960s and 1970s, encouraged once again by a liberal, optimistic spirit in American society (Diasio, 1971). Once again, people were convinced life could be made better for all. Occupational therapists increasingly took responsibility for transforming their discontent with the fragmentation that the reductionist mode of thinking carried with it. Efforts to see the larger whole of the persons we served led first to articulating human development as the theory base for the profession—the larger whole being understanding the person over the total life span as a basis for meeting patients' needs (Llorens, 1970, Mosey, 1968). Shortly thereafter came the articulation of the systems perspective as a theory base, which added to development a deeper appreciation of the role of the environment and of cognitive processes of purpose, goal, and choice (Diasio, 1967; Kielhofner & Burke, 1977, Howe & Briggs, 1982). The 1960s through the 1980s have been rich with many other formulations and expansions of theory by occupational therapists which will not be elaborated upon here. These have attempted to integrate occupational therapy practice around the perspective of a larger whole that can be served, based on theory development and scientific advancement.

REFLECTIONS ON A REDISCOVERED HERITAGE

It is indeed gratifying to see that the origins of thinking in occupational therapy are rooted in the emerging paradigm of the Systems Age, as well as saddening to think of the entropic effects of burnout and waste that resulted from the downswing cycles of Machine Age mentality which neglected so many aspects of patients' lives, and which undervalued contributions from professions such as occupational therapy. Dominant ideologies, containing the vision and purposes which direct resources in organizations and society, have had very real impacts on the quality of occupational therapy services that could be offered in any setting. Bockoven summarizes these cycles and their effects on the mental health arena:

> The significant point of interest in the history of American psychiatry is that the highest standards of care of the mentally ill . . . obtained when Americans lived in small communities, were inspired by a humanistic science and were motivated to go to the rescue of fellow men in distress. Conversely, the lowest standards of care obtained when Americans found themselves living in large industrial-urban communities, were awed by the authority of materialistic science and were motivated to get to the top in the competitive strife of rugged individualism. (p. 309)

An implicit decision about the division of labor between physicians and occupational therapists set the ongoing nurturance and evolution of the beliefs, philosophies, and principles, *outside* the boundaries of our own profession. The better trained physicians were assumed to supply these, while the action steps in implementation were left to the occupational therapists. Occupational therapists thus provided the pairs-of-hands (function) which were directed by another profession's (physicians) minds (will)—clearly an untenable position from which to evolve to full professional status. It is an irony of history that our origins in a way of thinking which emphasized mind-body unity would later unwittingly result in a division of labor in the professional arena that was characterized by an almost total mind-body split.

Decisions about the education of therapists stressed *function.* Johnson (1981) reflected on the implications this created for the profession. She described the early founders as having had "power created by belief and conviction, as they are honed by knowledge and observation; the power of disciplined minds and compassionate spirits" (p. 592). But then came an unspoken change:

> At this point an interesting turn occurred. Once OT was identified, demand for services quickly followed. The literature that I reviewed became silent about the scientific aspects of this great "discovery." . . . This growth was not accomplished without a price, however, and today we are beginning to pay that price. . . . Demands for service quickly increased and have continued unabated. There was little time for our founders' vision to be nurtured, expanded or understood intellectually or conceptually—rather, there was the demand that the ideas, the convictions, the values be put into action immediately. . . . Part of the price we now pay is that our directions frequently seem to be predicated not upon the observations and concepts of our founders but upon external sources and influences. . . . We have defined our problem as one of insufficient human resources at the entry level . . . rather than defining conceptual problems and perplexing questions. A theoretical framework cannot emerge from the problem of insufficient personnel. . . . The absence of well-defined theories limits our scope, our focus, and our research. . . . We need to recognize the value that knowledge, of itself, has, how it can support *all* of us, and how it can nurture and open doors for us. (pp. 592-597)

Thus the boundaries of the profession were set without the will component included within it. Yet, professionalism must come from *within* our own boundaries to be whole and to evolve. Furthermore, our state of *being,* or internal cohesion, as a profession will always be incomplete without the other two components; we will otherwise be adrift and without an identity around which we can define ourselves. *All three components of function, being, and will must be present within the profession's own boundaries to move in an evolutionary path forward.*

PLANNING FOR THE PATH FORWARD

Let us now return to our initial considerations about the great internal debate. Several major conclusions emerge from this review of our intellectual history.

1. The emerging premise of this paper is that, in view of enormously increasing environmental complexity, we must accelerate our professional path forward in delivering valued services to society by escalating our capacity to be thinkers as well as doers. In turbulent environments, where realities shift rapidly, it is easy to be reactive, to tend to the crisis at hand at the expense of the long-range perspective. Both now and in the future, we need a flexible, leadership-oriented, manager 'lly and clinically sophisticated membership who can ensu   lity in a world of increasingly scarce resources. Leader   n thinking (strategic planning, theory-building, and res   ) must come from *within* the boundaries of the profession.

2. Repe   we see that occupational therapy has shifted in direction   nphasis as a consequence of the way people were thinki   ir world view or paradigm. Similarly, the kind and qu   services given to the mentally ill were affected by the way   thought, both in prevalent paradigms of science and in   ral beliefs. These prevalent paradigms, which contain explicit   d implicit beliefs, philosophies and principles, direct people's efforts and have major impacts on the allocation of resources for specific services.

3. Great changes occurred for occupational therapists in the 1960s; during this period of expansion and optimism, we began to develop our own theories, always toward incorporating views of larger wholes (this occurred likewise in our practice with physical disabilities as we strove to understand patterns of movement rather than isolated ones, which occurred within an environmental context of gravity and other forces).

Our leadership's current search for the beliefs, philosophies, and principles to guide our practice is essential, for it builds and unifies our will as a profession. It is deeply related to enriching our understanding and creating a collective unity and vision about our fundamental purpose and contribution in society. It is on this foundation that long-range strategic thinking and planning for the future must build in our constant quest for higher standards of excellence in an ever-changing society. It is strongly related to what we must always keep in mind as we design our future and take action in our present (Ackoff, 1981, Clark, 1979). It is precisely the right place to start in transforming ourselves for the different challenges that will surely come in times ahead. It attempts to fill the gap that West so eloquently states: The mind of the profession. We cannot afford to leave this as a ''flat side'' of the profession; we cannot even *be* a full profession without a major allocation of our professional resources toward those ends. It is sad that we have paid such a heavy price for assuming that someone else out there will recognize and articulate our value to society; in that regard, we have done less for ourselves professionally in developing our minds, hearts, and hands than we routinely aspire to do for our clients or patients.

4. The profession's leaders are activating us to move toward developing theory and research. Practitioners, however, search primarily for more skills they can use on the job and hence restrain the allocation of resources the leaders would seek to deploy. *One way to reconcile these opposing forces is to develop a principle that both groups can deeply commit to and support.* I suggest that such a principle is: THE OCCUPATIONAL THERAPY PROFESSION IS COMMITTED TO CONTINUAL IMPROVEMENT OF ITS STANDARDS OF EXCELLENCE IN SERVICE TO OUR CLIENTS AND TO SOCIETY. Clearly, both sides of this debate hold this common theme. The *way* in which they hold that principle differs. Practitioners seek excellence and continuous improvement on the *operational* level of thinking, while leaders seek excellence in operational and also the *strategic* level of thinking. The strategic level of thinking looks further into the future and asks what kind of thinking needs to be in place to enhance our transformation into a fully sanctioned profession that readily articulates its service to society (Krone, 1984).

5. *Strategic allocation of our resources within the profession must occur* to develop the appropriate levels of personnel who can both articulate and appropriately expand the beliefs, philosophies, and principles of the profession, and demonstrate excellence in

practice, showing scientific evidence for their validity. There can be little doubt that these levels of personnel must have advanced study and education. If our history shows us anything, it shows us that *undereducated personnel at low levels in the organizational structure are unequal to the task of adequately advancing the vision of our founders.* Support for advanced study has been developing in the professional association, but not nearly at the pace demanded by constantly accelerating needs in organizations and in society for strategic thinkers. The rapid emergence of the new Systems Age paradigm resonates strongly with our founders' convictions; Buckley's *Modern Systems Research for the Behavioral Scientist* (1968) refers extensively back to the early work of Dewey and Mead, who contributed to our founders' visions of occupational therapy. These intellectual streams have lain dormant long enough; it is both our challenge and our opportunity to transcend our previous boundaries into new areas of intellectual discovery consonant with our past heritage.

6. Clearly, there are great cycles in these paradigms and in resulting services and programs, as is clearly evident both in occupational therapy and in mental health services. It might prove more useful to conceptualize these as alternative opportunities for expansion and concentration. Downswing cycles, particularly in the mental health arena where ideology so clearly continues to affect society's allocations of resources, need to be offset by the profession by consciously and strategically using these periods (which can continue for decades) for *concentrated work* on essentials in relevant arenas.

The current period in mental health, it seems, is in such a downswing, dominated now by the biological orientation of psychiatry and a societal lack of concern for the mentally ill in the name of cost containment. Despite evidence of the bankruptcy and failure of deinstitutionalization policies, tens of thousands of mentally ill are homeless in our cities. Once again we are seeing occupational therapy services being undervalued, despite emerging scientific evidence of its efficacy (Linn et al., 1979). It will be necessary to search assiduously for those pockets of excellence in practice, and bring them forward through in-depth studies. These periods are also times where extensive documentation through qualitative studies might eloquently give the disadvantaged a voice that can be heard. In every era, there has been some seminal book that has played a key role in reversing public opinion and arousing compassion for the less fortunate, such as Beers' *A Mind That Found Itself* (1908), and Deutsch's *Shame of the States* (1948). Could we, too, see ourselves as articulate advocates for improved services for the mentally ill and other neglected client and patient groups? Could we planfully allocate resources to those ends? The rewards could be multiple, with mutual benefit to patients, society, and ourselves.

7. Another aspect of our lost intellectual heritage that we are rediscovering is our roots in another research methodology, articulated and advanced by our early functionalist forerunners: that of qualitative research using naturalistic inquiry (Stryker, 1980). Although occupational therapists are increasingly advocating qualitative research, our graduate students are not exposed to its differing assumptions or paradigms, or its methodologies in traditional research courses. This is clearly an area where professional association leadership could pave the way for more widespread acceptance and use, especially since the inherent assumptions of qualitative research are closely aligned with both the emerging paradigms and theories, as well as with a clinical emphasis.

It is inescapably time for the highest quality of thinking to be brought to bear on our future development and transformation as a profession. That kind of organizing excellence will be required for us to fulfill the mandate from that ennobling vision of the past that enabled our birth as a profession. We will be measured by future generations by our consciousness in creating such opportunities and challenges for ourselves; we are both humbled and empowered by the inherent hazards in daring to be great.

REFERENCES

Ackoff, R. (1974) *Redesigning the Future.* New York: Wiley.
Ackoff, R. (1981) *Creating the Corporate Future.* New York: Wiley.
Ad Hoc Committee for Identifying the Philosophy of Occupational Therapy. (1977, October) *Occup. Ther. Newsletter,* 11.
Allen, A. & Cruickshank, D. (1977) Perceived problems of occupational therapists: A subset of the professional curriculum. *Am. J. Occup. Ther.,* 563.
Beer, S. (1975) *Platform for Change.* New York: Wiley, 24-37.
Beers, C. (1945) *A Mind that Found Itself.* Revised ed. Garden City, NY: Doubleday.
Bennett, J. (1978) *Deeper Man.* London: Turnstone Press.
Bennett, J. (1968) *The Dramatic Universe,* Vol. III. Sherborne, England: Coombe Springs Press.
Blauberg, I.V., Sadovsky, V.N., & Yudin, E.G. (1977) *Systems Theory: Philosophical and Methodological Problems.* Moscow: Progress Publishers.
Bing, R. (1981) Occupational Therapy Revisited: A paraphrastic journey. *Am. J. Occup. Ther.,* 35:499.

Bing, R. (1983) Beliefs at a new beginning. *Am. J. Occup. Ther.*, *37*:375.
Bockoven, J.S. (1963) *Moral treatment in American psychiatry.* New York: Springer.
Bohm, D. (1980) *Wholeness and the Implicate Order.* Routledge, Kegan Paul.
Buckley, W. (Ed.) (1968) *Modern Systems Research for the Behavioral Scientist.* Chicago: Aldine.
Burnham, W. (1924) *The Normal Mind.* New York: Appleton, 677.
Capra, F. (1982) *The Turning Point.* New York: Simon and Schuster.
Clark, J. (1978) New Patterns of Managerial Thinking. In Organizational Behavior Readings. San Jose.
Council on Education Committee to Review Educational Essentials. *Report of the Committee to Review Educational Essentials.* (1981) Rockville, MD: American Occupational Therapy Association.
Crampton, M. & Anderegg, G. (1961) Educational weaknesses and occupational stress. *Am. J. Occup. Ther.*, 233-241.
Deutsch, A. (1948) *Shame of the States.* New York: Harcourt Brace.
Dewey, J. The reflex arc concept in psychology. (1896) *Psychol. Rev.*, 357-370. Quoted in Slack, C. (1968) in "Feedback theory and the reflex arc concept," 317-320. *Modern Systems Research for the Behavioral Scientist*, Buckley, W. (ed.) Chicago: Aldine.
Diasio, K. (1970) The modern era: 1960-1970. *Am. J. Occup. Ther.*, *25*, 237-242.
Diasio, K. (1980) Occupational therapy in mental health: A time of challenge. *Occup. Ther. Ment. Hlth.*, *1*, 1-10.
Diasio, K. (1968) Psychiatric occupational therapy: Search for a conceptual framework in light of analytic ego psychology and learning theory. Also, Response by the author: On cybernetics, information processing, communication and systems theory. *Am. J. Occup. Ther.*, *22*, 400-414.
Diasio, K. (1981) Teaching systems thinking in a graduate professional school. In *General Systems Research and Design: Precursors and Futures*, Proceedings of the 25th Annual Meeting of the Society for General Systems Research. Louisville, KY: Society for General Systems Research. Reckmeyer, W. (ed.), 361-366.
Dunton, W. (1928) *Prescribing Occupational Therapy.* Springfield, IL.
Ferguson, M. (1980) *The Aquarian Conspiracy: Personal and Social Transformation in the 1980s.* Los Angeles: J.P. Tarcher.
Fidler, G. (1981) From crafts to competence. *Am. J. Occup. Ther.*, *35*, 567.
Fox, J. (1981) Occupational therapy theory development: Knowledge and values held by recent graduates. *Occup. Ther. J. Res.*, *1*, 79-93.
Guilfoyle, E. (1984) Eleanor Clarke Slagle Lectureship: Transformation of a profession. *Am. J. Occup. Ther.*, *38*, 575-584.
Harms. E. (1964) Beginnings of psychotherapy in America. *Am. J. Psychother.*, *18*, 287.
Heilbreder, E. (1973) Functionalism. In *Historical Conceptions of Psychology.* Henle, Mary; Jaynes, Julian; and Sullivan, John (Eds.) New York: Springer, 278-279.
Hospital and Library Service Bureau. (1925) *Bibliography on Occupational Therapy:* Jan. 1, 1895 to July 1, 1925. Chicago.
Howe, M. & Briggs, A. (1982) Ecological systems model for occupational therapy. *Am. J. Occup. Ther.*, *36*, 322.
James, W. (1892) *Psychology, Briefer Course.* Chapter 10, "Habit." New York: Holt, 134-150.
Johnson, J. (1981) Old values—new directions: Competence, adaptation, integration. *Am. J. Occup. Ther.*, *35*, 589.
Kanter, R. (1983) *The Changemasters.* New York: Simon and Schuster.
Kardiner, A. & Preble, E. (1961) *They Studied Man.* New York: Mentor.
Kielhofner, G. & Burke, J. (1977) Occupational therapy after 60 years: An account of changing identity and knowledge. *Am. J. Occup. Ther.*, *31*, 675.
Kielhofner, G. & Burke, J. (1980) A model of human occupation, Part 1. Conceptual framework and content. *Am. J. Occup. Ther.*, *34*, 572.
Kielhofner, G. (Ed.) (1983) *Health through Occupation: Theory and Practice in Occupational Therapy.* Philadelphia: F.A. Davis.

Krone, C. (1983-1984) *Strategic Series Seminars.* Carmel, CA.

Kubie, L. (1960) *The Riggs Story.* New York: Hoebart Press, 57, 85.

Kuhn, Thomas. (1962) *The Structure of Scientific Revolutions.* Chicago: University of Chicago Press.

Lief, A. (1948) *The Commonsense Psychiatry of Adolf Meyer.* New York: McGraw-Hill.

Linn, M., Coffey, E. et al. (1979) Day treatment and psychotropic drugs in the aftercare of schizophrenic patients. *Arch. Gen. Psychiat. 36,* 1055-1066.

Llorens, L. (1970) Facilitating growth and development: The promise of occupational therapy. *Am. J. Occup. Ther., 24,* 93, 1970.

Maxwell, J.D. & Maxwell, M.P. (1978) *Occupational Therapy: The Diffident Profession.* Kingston, Ontario: Queens University.

Meyer, A. (1922) The philosophy of occupation therapy. *Arch. Occ. Ther., 1,* 1.

Mosey, A. (1968) Recapitulation of ontogenesis: A theory for practice of occupational therapy. *Am. J. Occup. Ther., 22,* 426.

Muncie, W. (1939) *Psychobiology and Psychiatry: A Textbook.* St. Louis: C.V. Mosby, 23-24.

Musto, D. (1975) Short history of orthopsychiatry. In *Mental Health and Social Change.* New York: AMS Press, 6.

Peacock, A.C. & O'Shea, B. (1984) *Am. J. Occup. Ther., 38,* 517-521.

Radonsky, V. (1980) Personality characteristics of the published and nonpublished occupational therapist. *Am. J. Occup. Ther., 34,* 208-212.

Report of the Mental Health Task Force. (September, 1976) *Occupational Ther. Newspaper, 30,* 6-7.

Report of the Ad Hoc Committee on Education. (1978) In Nationally speaking: Issues in education. *Am. J. Occup. Ther., 32,* 355-358.

Reilly, M. (1962) Occupational therapy can be one of the great ideas of twentieth century medicine. *Am. J. Occup. Ther., 16,* 1.

Rogers, J. & Mann, W. (1980) The relationship between professional productivity and educational level, part 2. *Am. J. Occup. Ther., 34,* 460-468.

Schultz, D. (1960) *A History of Modern Psychology.* New York: Academic Press.

Sicherman, B. (1975) The New Psychiatry: Medical and behavioral Science, 1895-1921. In *American Psychoanalysis: Origins and Development:* The Adolf Meyer Seminar. Q., Jacques, and Carlson, E., eds. New York: Brunner Mazel, 20-37.

Stryker, S. (1980) *Symbolic Interactionism,* Menlo Park, CA: Benjamin/Cummings.

West, W. (1978) Historical perspectives. In *Occupational Therapy, 2001.* American Occupational Therapy Association: Rockville, MD.

Woodside, H. (1970) The development of occupational therapy: 1910-1929. *Am. J. Occup. Ther., 25,* 226-230, 229.

Adolf Meyer
and the Development
of American Psychiatry

Theodore Lidz

ABSTRACT. Adolf Meyer was a major force in molding psychiatry into its current form; his teachings are so solidly incorporated into American psychiatric theory and practice that the extent of his influence is often overlooked. He brought American psychiatry its pluralistic and instrumental orientation, its holistic approach, its psychobiological understanding that human behavior is integrated at a symbolic level, its conceptualization of psychiatric disorders as maladaptive reaction patterns rather than as discrete disease entities, its interest in the psychotherapy of the psychoses. He provided psychiatry with a fundamental scientific orientation that fitted into the remainder of science and also opened the way for the inclusion of data concerning human experience and biography in biological thinking.

On a similar occasion, the celebration of the 80th birthday of his teacher August Forel in 1929, Adolf Meyer said: "Next to the interrelationships between parents and children, the association between teacher and pupil is potentially the most important in the development of a civilization." Those of us who worked with him in the Phipps Clinic; who listened and puzzled over what he meant; who came under the compelling influence of his magnetic personality, his humanism, and of his intellect and vast erudition are apt to feel that Adolf Meyer is still very much with us. As a great teacher he

Dr. Lidz is with the Department of Psychiatry, Yale University School of Medicine, 333 Cedar Street, New Haven, CT. Until recently he was also with the Center for Advanced Study in the Behavioral Sciences, Stanford, CA.

Read as the Adolf Meyer Lecture on the occasion of the Adolf Meyer centenary at the 122nd annual meeting of the American Psychiatric Association, Atlantic City, NJ, May 9-13, 1966. The lecture was made possible through the support of Smith, Kline and French Laboratories.

This article originally appeared in *The American Journal of Psychiatry*, Vol. 123:3, pp. 320-332, September 1966. It is being reprinted with permission of the American Psychiatric Association.

has become a part of his pupils. If the terms were not somewhat inappropriate to the occasion, I might say that some of his thinking has become part of our ego functioning, and his presence survives in our superegos.

However, for most psychiatrists Adolf Meyer has become little more than a name: an honored and even a revered name—though they may be uncertain why. Of course, he is the founder of psychobiology, but what does this term that is defined so variously really mean? And he fostered a system of classification that used such outrageous Greek derivatives as "hyperthyrmergasia" and "pareregasia," which some continue to learn for the board examinations.

The reasons for his position are not readily learned from his writings. Although he could write lucidly and forcefully when presenting a critique of a mental hospital system or a plan for psychiatric education, most of his theoretic papers are illuminating only to those who already know the gist of his thinking. One searches in vain for case reports of patients similar to those stylistic masterpieces in Freud's writings. No, when I have borrowed the volumes of his collected papers from the Yale and Stanford libraries, the bindings still crackled when opened and the pages were crisp and virginal, unblemished by pencil.

Despite the limited appreciation of the nature of Meyer's contributions, I believe that his influence remains very much alive: not only in his students but in virtually all American psychiatrists. It enters into the way in which we talk to our patients and conceptualize their problems; in how we think about personality development and the nature of psychiatric disorders; and, indeed, in why we are interested in the person and his life experiences rather than, like so many of our continental colleagues, primarily in a disease process.

However, his major contributions to psychiatric thought were made prior to World War I, which seemed the remote past when he retired in 1941 at the age of 75. His failure to develop and specify more precisely his own orientation or to develop a new synthesis with psychoanalytic teachings seemed to be retarding progress. His commanding influence and his critical ways seemed binding and restrictive to his students, who filled a large proportion of the chairs of psychiatry. Most of Meyer's contributions had by then become so solidly incorporated into the body of American psychiatry that they seemed self-evident. Doubts were expressed that he had ever made any substantial original contributions.

It is my thesis that Adolf Meyer was not only the dominant figure in American psychiatry between 1895 and 1940, but one of the two great figures who changed psychiatry into a dynamic therapy and into a discipline that affords meaningful insights into human behavior; and that he was the person largely responsible for the pragmatic, instrumental, and pluralistic approach that has been distinctive of American psychiatry. The remarkable development of American psychiatry during the past 25 years has often been attributed to the leavening influence of psychoanalysis. However, psychoanalysis rapidly found a place in medical teaching and thought in this country that it never achieved in its European birthplace; and psychoanalysis changed considerably in its transplantation. In contrast to other countries, American psychiatry had achieved a genetic dynamic approach prior to the impact of psychoanalysis because of Meyer and his teachings.

The direction that psychiatry has taken in the United States is to some degree a cultural matter. Psychiatric perspectives are always closely related to a culture's basic philosophy and its concepts of the nature of man. A new and rapidly changing country was not to be bound by beliefs in the hereditary determination of character. The personality traits of its people changed from generation to generation and sometimes in the same generation when a person found a new and more hospitable environment,* in contrast to European communities where sons generally followed fathers in occupation, status, and character traits.

The American was often in a position that made him conscious of how greatly differences in cultural heritages contributed to differences in personality characteristics. Such influences could not but affect the orientation of American psychiatry. The basic approach may have been attained without Adolf Meyer, for it seems indigenous. The wheel seems obvious too, but it was only invented once. If Meyer was not the father of the approach, he was certainly the accoucheur, the preceptor, the goad.

AMERICAN PSYCHIATRY IN THE 1890s

To understand the force and sweep of Meyer's impact upon the course of American psychiatry, we must seek to peer through the

---

*The changes in Kurt Weill's music and George Grosz's painting after they came to the United States from Germany are patent examples.

veil of three-quarters of a century to gain a glimpse of the psychiatric scene in the early 1890s. Fortunately, Meyer's incisive report in 1894 to the Governor of Illinois on the treatment of the insane helps re-create the situation.[13]

The period of moral treatment of insanity, when hospitals were small and the superintendents knew and spoke with each patient daily, had passed. Already in 1870, John P. Gray, the dean of American alienists and head of the Utica State Hospital, was proud of having eliminated all "moral and mental" cause of insanity from his statistics because the "mind cannot become diseased, but only the brain."

Starting in the mid-19th century, the advances in microscopic pathology, the discoveries of specific bacterial causes of diseases, and particularly the isolation of general paresis as an entity caused by syphilis, led to a search for similar tangible causes for all mental disorders. Following the lead of Kahlbaum and Hecker, efforts were made to define specific disease entities, whose causes would then be found in some pathology and dysfunction of the brain cells. The clergy with their moral and spiritual concerns had been vanquished in the fight over Darwinism, and human experiences which had no tangible existence in the body were not a topic for scientific study, but were the province of the novelist.

The problems extended beyond medicine and science into the social orientation of the period. Industrialization and geographic expansion had created an elite of vast wealth and masses of impoverished and exploited proletarians. Social Darwinism furnished a useful philosophy. Life was a struggle for survival, and the unfit must be weeded out to make room for the more capable: it would strengthen the nation. Perhaps social Darwinism reinforced the Protestant ethic, particularly Calvinist predetermination; but now one proved oneself a member of the elect by outwitting, outfighting, and outclimbing others. Evolution and particularly social Darwinism had often been perverted into a doctrine of "devil take the hindmost" and a justification of the entrenched hierarchy.

With the rapid industrialization and accompanying urbanization and massive immigration, mental hospitals grew unwieldy, eliminating the possibility of personal attention to patients, even if it were considered worthwhile. Hospitals deteriorated and humanism in psychiatry declined.

Further, there were few psychiatrists outside of institutions.

There were no real training programs for psychiatrists; if psychiatry had a place in the medical school curriculum anywhere, it consisted of little more than the demonstration of some cases. Mental hospitals provided custodial care, and it is apparent from Clifford Beers' account[1] that the care even in private institutions was devoid of understanding, callous, and often brutal.

Psychiatry and psychiatrists lacked purpose and direction. They classified and they provided shelter, often under conditions that insured a grave prognosis, and they waited for someone to find the cause of these diseases. The research-minded peered at gross and microscopic specimens of brains, or pursued the relatively simple chemistry and physiology of the period in search of direction.

Adolf Meyer entered into this situation, saw the need, saw a way, and became the man. Within a few short years he provided a new orientation and stimulated his colleagues into renewed activity. He insisted that the patients' life experiences were pertinent to etiology and provided guides to treatment, and that interest in the physiological must fit into study of the total pattern of a person's current behavior and its biographical origins: a genetic-dynamic approach to mental disorders. He understood that human behavior can only be comprehended properly through study of its integration at the symbolic level—his psychobiological orientation, which overcame the mind-brain parallelism that had stifled thought and thwarted research concerning mental problems.

He combatted the "neurologizing" of psychiatry, the pessimistic inertia that made the term "dementia praecox" a sentence to a living death rather than a diagnosis, and opposed the Kraepelinian concepts of discrete disease entities of organic or hereditary etiology. Above all, he knew what needed to be taught and devoted himself to teaching a coherent and useful approach to understanding human behavior.

What had happened? How did this 27-year-old Swiss neuropathologist, essentially untrained in psychiatry, come to exert such profound influence so rapidly? According to Zilboorg and Henry in their *History of Medical Psychology*[25], Meyer introduced the best tradition of European psychiatry into the American scene. This is a gross misapprehension for, as I shall elaborate, he introduced a uniquely American orientation into psychiatry, an approach that was also in the process of transforming American education. Its essence lies in the belief that through the use of human intellect, ingenuity, and effort the face of nature, even human nature, can be modified and man's adaptive capacities broadened and improved.

A COMMON SENSE CULTURAL HERITAGE

I had long been puzzled—since I first met Adolf Meyer and recognized the similarity of his teachings to those of James and Dewey—how it happened that a Swiss had embraced pragmatism, indeed, had found in it his natural voice. Most Europeans trained in the German philosophical tradition not only have difficulty in grasping the importance of these American philosophers but are apt to be contemptuous of them and their practical and nonmetaphysical approach. For a long time, I had thought that as the Swiss are eminently practical and democratic, Adolf Meyer as a Swiss intellectual had fitted into the American way of thinking.

Fortunately Manfred Bleuler was also puzzled and as a Swiss did not attribute Meyer's outlook to his Swiss education. He investigated Meyer's family background and discovered that Adolf Meyer's grandfather had been a follower of an eighteenth century Swiss folk philosopher, Jakob Gujer, better known as Kleinjogg or Little Joe. The Meyer family had intermarried with the Gujers, eventually purchased their farm, and considered themselves the spiritual heirs of the Kleinjogg tradition.

Kleinjogg had practiced and taught an instrumental approach to farming, observing what worked and what did not work, and trying out new ways that seemed to make sense rather than blindly following tradition, as did other peasants. He fostered communal activity and teamwork. At first he was hated and considered a menace for departing from ways that had become sacred through long usage; but when his techniques bore results he became a revered and widely renowned person whom Goethe, Pestalozzi, and other great men visited. Kleinjogg's basic concerns were with how people could be healthy and happy. He demonstrated that joy could be obtained from useful work and the ensuing accomplishment, and he emphasized that children became happy and skillful adults only through the example of parents. Harmony between parents was the highest good.[2]

Of course, it required more than a family tradition to permit the synthesis of ideas that occurred in Adolf Meyer. He followed the path of his physician uncle rather than that of his father, a Zwinglian minister; he once suggested that his uncle and father represented body and mind, the division which he had to resolve.

The reasons are not clear why Meyer turned to France, England, and Scotland rather than to Germany and Austria to supplement his medical education. Perhaps he was drawn to British empiricism or the great neurological schools of London and Edinburgh; but the move was felicitous, for in England he encountered two decisive influences. Unhappy with the Swiss and German physiological approach to medicine that neglected the total human organism and its adaptation, he was attracted to Thomas Huxley's biological orientation. Huxley, a good Darwinian, studied how the total organism fitted in with the environment—an ecological approach—and he also taught that science consisted of the application of trained common sense.

Meyer also came under the influence of Hughlings Jackson, who applied Spencer's philosophy to bring order into the understanding of the functioning of the central nervous system. Jackson's theories of the evolution and dissolution of the central nervous system suggested Meyer's segmental-suprasegmental approach to neuroanatomy. But even more important, Jackson's concepts of levels of integration prepared the way for the basic psychobiological concept that human behavior is integrated at the symbolic level. These influences would take time to crystallize.

After completing his thesis on the forebrain of reptiles under Forel's supervision and receiving his doctorate, Meyer failed to gain the university position he sought. Not wishing to become a practitioner, he decided to make his way in the United States. He hoped to find a post at one of the three exciting new centers at the Johns Hopkins, Clark, and Chicago universities. Unsuccessful, he decided to move to Chicago where he knew a promising young neurologist.* He would eventually gain posts in all three of these universities.

EARLY YEARS IN THE MIDWEST

Meyer started a neurological practice in Chicago in 1892, but in the following year gladly accepted the post as pathologist at the new Kankakee State Hospital to pursue his dominant neuropathological and neuroanatomical interests. He had not considered becoming a psychiatrist despite his studies with Forel, in part because he

---

*H. H. Donaldson, whom Meyer had met when he studied with von Monakow and whom he again met in London just before sailing for the United States.

believed it required a facility in verbal communication which he lacked.

At Kankakee he taught the staff neuroanatomy and neuropathology but found his interests shifting to the living. He had a new motivation. He believed that his emigration had helped precipitate his widowed mother's severe depression. His mother had the fixed delusion that he was dead, and he grasped the meaningfulness of the delusion. He had always considered his mother eminently sensible and sane, but Forel considered her condition hopeless. Perhaps her recovery, despite the great psychiatrist's prognosis, contributed to Meyer's skepticism about disease entities and his aversion for grave prognostications.

He became interested in talking to patients about their lives and found that they seemed to explain much of why they had become ill. He was developing dynamic concepts of the importance of childhood experiences. In a paper written in 1895, he admonished that hereditary factors could be overemphasized, as children of abnormal parents are "exposed from birth to acquire unconsciously habits of a morbid character."[14] He was turning into a psychiatrist.

However, something outside of the hospital probably had a decisive effect upon the development of this young man for whom "the problem of the nature of man—of mind and body and their integration—was not a mere abstract problem."[16] He was introduced to the writings of Charles Peirce and William James by Paul Carus** and became friends with John Dewey, and later with George H. Mead and Charles Cooley. He found himself caught up in one of the most exciting phases of American intellectual history. His friendship with Dewey would be renewed in New York ten years later and have a still more pervasive influence. I believe that Meyer now found answers to many of his philosophical preoccupations and doubts: solutions that had a profound and practical effect upon his thought and beliefs and would serve as a guide for his activities.

There are repeated references in Meyer's writings to the importance of Peirce, James, and Dewey to his development. It is difficult to know which ideas he gained from these kindred spirits and how much their ideas gave him confidence to elaborate his own concepts. The resultant synthesis, however it came about, enabled Meyer to move decisively into action.

**The philosophic publisher of *The Monist,* and the founder of The Open Court Press, which published inexpensive, reliable issues of philosophic classics.

Meyer found that these philosophers, particularly Peirce, took an unequivocal stand against Cartesian concepts of a self-contained "mind" unrelated to a body, a person, and the person's needs and desires; against a mind capable of finding an ultimate "truth" through the exertion of pure reason. Man is part of nature and, having evolved in relation to his environment, his sense organs are formed to help him adapt in nature. His mind is not something abstract and discrete from his body but is intensely practical. Man is unique in being able to think, and thought is his chief tool of adaptation, his chief means of extricating himself from predicaments, for reshaping and altering things in the environment, of moving toward future ends rather than simply being impelled by his body's needs.

Indeed, Peirce could not conceive of thought divorced from circumstances that created problems requiring solution. Truth is not a platonic abstraction, but something to be gained from experience—that is, through experiment. We can only know what we experience, and consequently experience must be a valid subject for scientific study. Experiment is not something confined to a laboratory, but is man's way of guiding himself into the future—or at least it can be if he gives up superstition and blind adherence to authority and custom. Meyer was certainly reminded of the common sense wisdom of Kleinjogg.

The purpose of thinking—of the mind—is not the satisfaction of idle intellectual curiosity, nor the pursuit of an ideal good in seeking after the "truth." The role of mentation is to direct one's life and to help change the world if necessary. Thought is not the antithesis of action; it is a type of action. It is a way of imaginatively trying out alternatives before committing oneself to irrevocable action. It is imaginative trial and error, a kind of experimental maneuver. Ideas are important, for they are plans of action. What we believe and think determines what we do, and for ideas to be effective they must be related to human needs and provoke human will.

The mind or intelligence exists as a problem-solving power, but one does not gain the secrets of nature and learn to control nature either by observation alone or by reasoning alone. The principles by which nature operates yield to inquiry insofar as we intervene and try out various alternatives: try out what works and what does not work. Dewey insisted that in order to discover answers, one had to place questions. More specifically, through devising experimental situations that asked these questions through activity, we literally force nature to yield its secrets.

The essence of pragmatic, pluralistic thinking is that through the ingenuity, thought, and effort of man, the face of nature can be altered to man's needs. Such concepts stand at the core of the American tradition. Such ideas obviously turn away from the idea of a completed world which man seeks to know so that he can fit himself into it, or ideas of a given truth we must uncover, or even of those evolutionary concepts which maintain that everything unrolls in a predetermined and irrevocable manner.

Meyer clearly believed that we humans are capable of the eminently practical task of reshaping the world and transforming ourselves. Our actions depend upon decision, and decision means using judgment in selecting what is relevant and rejecting or neglecting the irrelevant. Each decision means taking one course and neglecting the other potentialities. In areas where decisions are vital, the inability to reach a decision is decision through default. Therefore, when no other guides are available, we have the right to follow our beliefs. Indeed, as James pointed out, a willingness to act on belief can sometimes create the fact.

Thus, only if Adolf Meyer acted on his unproven belief that schizophrenic patients could be helped through altering their milieu and modifying their habits of thinking could the fact be demonstrated. Belief should be based upon experience, and James not only considered it a person's right to take his own experience seriously, but his obligation to do so and use it to guide his beliefs, thoughts, and actions.

These philosophers were not concerned with ideas for the sake of ideas or as guides to eternal salvation, which could continue forever and make little difference except to foster scholastic argumentation and displays of intellectual brilliance. As ideas were guides to action, it became essential to select topics that made a difference in solving problems of living. Perhaps of great importance to the young Adolf Meyer was to have such confirmation "that steering clear of useless puzzles liberates a mass of new energy." He found a new freedom, as if the old world and its weighty traditional and unresolvable philosophies had been taken off his back. He was ready to transform the face of psychiatry.

The life stories of patients seemed to make sense; their experiences seemed to clarify why they were disturbed and suggested ways of helping them. Bolstered by pragmatism, he could cease looking for "something else" to explain their mental disorders. As a neuroanatomist and neuropathologist, he knew that what he found in a brain might explain disorganization of thought and behavior, but it could never explain a life story or show how to remedy it. He grasped the need for a genetic-dynamic understanding of mental disorders in terms of the unique biography of each individual. He had the right to trust his common sense and he taught his colleagues to trust theirs.

The meaning of Meyer's common sense psychiatry has often been misunderstood. He was not advocating that psychiatrists rely upon naive common sense: he devoted much of his life to teaching the uncommon sense provided by training and experience. What he meant was that psychiatrists must be willing to use data about a patient's life in its own terms, not persist in seeking something behind and beyond experiences. He had found psychiatrists neglecting the obvious, the "common sense," because the scientific tradition insisted that they must seek causes in the brain cells, physiology, or biochemistry; or because they must cure the "mind" that they could not locate rather than seek to modify the patient's life and behavior.

Eventually, I believe after his association with Dewey in New York, he would teach his pupils to regard each patient as an "experiment in nature," one of his most felicitous phrases. The observer could scrutinize life stories for what seemed to make a difference and search out common developmental factors in patients with similar difficulties. The therapist's interventions could then be considered attempts to alter the course of the specific experiment of nature.

If so much of what man does depends on what he believes and thinks, it seemed essential to consider just how thinking affects man's total functioning, including his bodily functioning. Meyer saw the way to overcome the age-old conflict between physiological and psychological concepts of man and to open the way for eradicating the body-mind dichotomy, or the brain-mind parallelism.

The conception of psychobiological integration is Meyer's major contribution, and because of lack of understanding of its core concept and its ramifications, it has not been fully appreciated. Human behavior is integrated through mentation; what man thinks affects his functioning down to a cellular level, and his symbolizations are critical to his functioning as a social organism. Lower levels of integration, physical, chemical, cellular, physiologic, etc., are obviously important and require study; they can influence symbolic activity, but one can never study or understand what is uniquely and essentially human by studying these lower levels of integration.

Problems of human adaptation and maladaptation and man's functioning as an integrated unit must be studied at the psychobiological level.

MASSACHUSETTS AND EARLY FAME

After but two short years, Meyer left Kankakee for the Worcester State Hospital and Clark University. Though he again started as a neuropathologist he had been promised a wider scope. The neuropathologist had turned psychopathologist, for he felt that the pathology of mental disorders could only be found in the living. Soon he was clinical director, for his teaching about patients had turned Worcester into a major training center for psychiatrists.

By the close of the 1890s, Meyer, despite his youth, was already a famous person, so that when he took a firm stand against Kraepelin's 1896 nosology which considered mental disorders as specific disease entities it was a decisive step for American psychiatry. Virtually everywhere else the concept of disease entities was accepted and served as a focus for the search for specific physical etiologies. Instead, Meyer taught that the various disorders were different reaction patterns, differences that depended on constitution and life experiences. They were, in essence, the different ways in which people manifested their incapacities to adapt successfully. Eventually, he used the term *ergasia* (based on the Greek root for "work") to designate mentally integrated activity, and developed a terminology of the ergasias to designate the major reaction patterns. He was seeking to get away from the connotation of specific diseases inherent in the conventional Kraepelinian nosology.

Although Meyer did not disregard the potential importance of unknown hereditary factors, he refused to accept the prevalent pessimism about combatting hereditary conditions. Pragmatically he focused on what could be worked with—change the environment, alter habit patterns and ways of thinking, help the patient solve or resolve problems. See what works and what does not work; mobilize the patient's assets, and they may suffice to counterbalance his deficiencies. Meyer was a meliorist, interested in improvement when he could not cure; and he taught that every patient should somehow be better off because of his relationship to the psychiatrist.

Meyer then applied the same concept of reaction types to schizophrenia. Mental disorders are different ways of reacting, each somewhat individual and never a clear-cut entity. As what one thinks and believes directs much of one's behavior, it seemed perfectly feasible to Meyer that the bizarre behavior of the schizophrenic could be due to deteriorations of habits of thinking* and behaving rather than to some deterioration or dysfunction of the brain. A person was schizophrenic or manifested a parergasic reaction; he never "had schizophrenia."

Meyer promulgated such ideas as early as 1905, and in 1909 at the famous 20th anniversary celebration of Clark University where Freud gave his five lectures on psychoanalysis, Meyer's address was "A Dynamic Interpretation of Dementia Praecox." Meyer stood virtually alone in maintaining the potentiality that schizophrenia could be a psychogenic condition, disappointed that Eugen Bleuler and Jung considered the psychological manifestations they described and studied so effectively as secondary to some toxic condition affecting the brain.

It was largely Meyer's influence that made the psychotherapeutic treatment of schizophrenia an American idiosyncrasy. Sullivan, in the 1920s, took heart in his early therapeutic efforts from Meyer's orientation, and Meyer encouraged Kempf in the first psychoanalyses of hospitalized schizophrenic patients. The convergence of Meyer's influence, Sullivan's insights, and later, the work of Lewis Hill and Frieda Fromm-Reichmann, made the Baltimore-Washington area almost the only place in the world where serious psychotherapy of schizophrenic patients was practiced before World War II.

In 1902 Meyer became chief of the Pathological Institute of the New York State hospitals, accepting the position under the proviso that the Institute move to the Manhattan State Hospital where there were patients. He had transformed Worcester State Hospital into a real training center and he now had the opportunity to revitalize and improve the entire New York system of 13 institutions.

He proceeded to conduct intensive week-long sessions in each hospital, teaching his clinical approach, his emphasis upon the history and mental status, and the utilization of the patient's assets. The old nosology was discarded. He was not concerned with a mind divorced from a body but in the person in a concrete setting seeking to cope with his experiences. Psychiatry could try to help patients to

---

*"Habit" for Meyer had the broad connotation of organized patterns of behavior and thinking, much as Peirce used the word.

achieve more workable and useful solutions to problems, and it could seek to modify the circumstances in which they lived. Meyer had brought a new young wife with him to New York, and to help him learn more about patients' family settings and to help modify them, Mrs. Mary Brooks Meyer became the first psychiatric social worker, continuing until the state system brought professionals to the task.

Dr. Meyer had given considerable thought to the need for more active public interest in the mentally ill; to ways of rallying support for the hospitals; and to the pressing need for preventive work—as can be noted in his earliest psychiatric papers concerned with children and the prophylactic opportunities in the school system. When Clifford Beers came to him with the manuscript of *A Mind That Found Itself*[1] and plans to form an organization to improve hospitals, Meyer convinced this ardent man to found an organization with broader and more prophylactic objectives. Meyer suggested the name "Mental Hygiene Movement" and assured Beers of strong professional support.

Meyer welcomed psychoanalysis as another genetic dynamic psychiatry that was interested in the individual and his development. Although from his first contacts with analysis he had reservations and misgivings, he drew attention to its strengths—to the concept of substitutive reactions, to the importance of the scientific scrutiny of sexual behavior, and particularly to Freud's emphasis on the importance of early childhood. Soon after Freud's Clark lectures, Meyer introduced Freud's ideas to a conference of New York state hospital physicians and became one of the founding members of the New York and the American Psychoanalytic Associations. Meyer's genetic dynamic orientation as well as his early interest prepared the way for the acceptance of analysis in academic psychiatric circles in the United States in striking contrast to Europe. In Europe, analysis stood in direct opposition to the brain mythology and disease entity approach and was scorned by the professors as unscientific "*Quatsch,*" but in this country the critical battle concerning the pertinence of personality development and experience had been fought and won by Meyer, who was becoming the foremost American psychiatrist.

A DECISIVE EFFECT ON MEDICAL EDUCATION

Indeed, in 1908, when the Johns Hopkins Medical School decided to build a psychiatric unit, Adolf Meyer was the obvious and unanimous choice for the professorship. Before he left New York he started the city's first psychiatric outpatient clinic at Cornell, and had the name of the Pathologic Institute changed to the New York State Psychiatric Institute, once again emphasizing the need to study and work with the living.

Johns Hopkins offered the opportunities he sought: to introduce psychobiology and dynamic psychiatry into the medical school curriculum—at that time, into *the* medical school; to establish a university training center for psychiatrists; to bring psychiatry into a close working relationship with the remainder of medicine; to build and develop a university psychiatric research and teaching hospital; to organize and run a model psychiatric hospital that was community-oriented. As this phase of Meyer's activities is well known, I shall not expand on how he achieved these objectives, which had a crucial impact upon American medicine and psychiatry. These activities consumed his time and energy, for he was a perfectionist. The medical school program, the residency training, the facilities, and the treatment program of the Phipps Clinic provided the standards for other medical schools and institutions for the next 25 years.

A measure of a teacher can be found in his pupils. I shall not name individuals, but a large proportion of the chairs of psychiatry have been filled by his students; many texts of psychiatry, child psychiatry, and public health psychiatry issued from their minds and pens. His students have carried out some of the most significant psychiatric research of the past half-century. Because Meyer had students and not disciples, they have not always adhered to his psychobiology but almost always a good deal has remained of Meyer's basic orientation and his attitudes toward patients.

How is it then that psychiatrists trained since World War II—over 75 percent of our psychiatrists—know so little about Meyer's contributions? The reasons are complex. What he taught was not dramatic, and much had been incorporated into the core of psychiatric teachings. Then, as pluralistic and instrumental thinking pervaded our educational system, much of what Meyer had initiated seemed simply common sense, just as he had wished. It became necessary to go to Europe to realize how differently psychiatrists could conceptualize the nature of man and mental disorders, and Americans no longer went abroad to study psychiatry.

The disinterest also was due to the fact that Meyer had not taught a system of psychiatry but an approach. He spent too much of his own life in overcoming philosophical systems that had blocked constructive thinking. He wished his students to think for themselves and gradually build upon firm foundations. He knew that he did not possess final answers.

However, Meyer had difficulty in generalizing. He could always think of the exceptions and see alternative ideas. He tended to emphasize the individuality of the patient and his development. He sought after similarities in the histories and behavior of patients with related reaction patterns but they were of broad dimensions. He did not, for example, outline developmental stages and their critical tasks; nor did he focus upon essential developmental themes that are significant to all lives. In brief, he did not provide organizing constructs and abstractions that are essential to the progress of science and necessary to provide reference points for understanding patients and conducting psychotherapy.

There were, of course, aspects of psychoanalysis that he could have included in the psychobiological approach. Psychoanalysis also provides genetic dynamic understanding of patients, and it is concerned with behavior integrated through symbolic functioning. Meyer's early hopes for such fusion dissipated for reasons that seem clear enough. Freud's emphasis on the primacy of unconscious motivation and his attempts to adhere to strict determinism run counter to the instrumentalist belief that thinking is a major adaptive technique that can change the course of events.* The assured emphasis that human motivation could be traced to vicissitudes of the libidinal and aggressive drives seemed to neglect other obvious influences. But Meyer particularly objected to what seemed to him the complex and premature systematization of analysis which became increasingly complex because of its prematurity. Further, Meyer did not properly grasp the nature of the transference relationship either as a therapeutic lever or as a means of focusing biographical data.** He had difficulty understanding why the personality study or the distributive analysis that he taught and which were aimed primarily at providing intellectual insights were not adequate.

Psychotherapy is a difficult and elusive activity, and psychiatrists seek clear-cut and definite answers, guidelines, and rules. Meyer

---

*Freud, however, was seeking to make the unconscious become conscious to permit rational, reality-oriented thinking; and he was overstating the determinism when he really wished to emphasize that mental activity was not something separate from the body, as biological drives strongly influence thought and behavior. He also showed that through understanding of unconscious processes, more of behavior could be understood as dependent upon previous experiences.

**An opinion derived from personal discussions with Dr. Meyer.

could not offer such answers. Psychoanalysis was willing to provide answers and specific directions. The influx of excellent psychoanalytic teachers from Europe just at the time of Meyer's retirement helped propel psychoanalysis to the front of the psychiatric scene.* Psychobiology was eclipsed even though, as we have seen, it continued to exert a very active influence upon American psychiatry, including psychoanalytic thinking.

MEYER'S CONTRIBUTION: A NEW ORIENTATION

Perhaps Meyer's job was done. He had accomplished a great deal, nurturing and shaping American psychiatry through its formative years, and now it was time for a new era. Quite aside from the attractiveness of psychoanalysis, there were serious limitations to psychobiology. Meyer had been primarily concerned with the mind-body unity and the integration of the individual. He had stopped with his important realization that human behavior is integrated through mentation. Psychobiology in this form did not do much to clarify the importance of cultural and social factors in human integration. Meyer focused upon integration at a symbolic level, behavior integrated through mentation. It is necessary to focus upon that other aspect of symbolic functioning—communication—to increase the range and comprehension of psychobiology. Man depends upon verbal communication as well as upon its internal counterpart, thought, for his adaptation. Through communicating what he learns he has gradually built up cultures and become dependent upon learning and using the techniques of his culture to survive and adapt. The family is the basic transmitter of the culture's language, techniques, roles, and institutions to each new generation. Man has two heritages—a biological and a cultural—and it is necessary to understand their interrelationship and fusion to achieve a general "field" theory, or comprehensive working theory for the study of human development and maldevelopment.**

---

*These European-trained teachers had little if any appreciation of the American intellectual tradition and the pragmatic pluralistic approach that its psychiatry had taken, which may well have led to disregard of a basic component—albeit an almost unexpressed component—of Meyer's teachings and also to some of the problems of deviance from classic analysis in the United States. Moreover, in Germanic countries the pupil is supposed to learn and accept what the teacher teaches.

**Such expansion or reorganization of psychobiology has been further amplified in my essays, *The Family and Human Adaptation.*[10]

Meyer was prepared to fade from the scene, to be supplanted by others and have his ideas enter into the unexpressed foundations of psychiatry. He said:

> We see ourselves as organisms . . . that . . . do their best under the idea of making themselves unnecessary through their achievements. . . . We do not . . . aspire to eternity, but to leave . . . the best opportunity for new times and new life. So it is with me. The goal of medicine is peculiarly the goal of making itself unnecessary: of influencing life so that what is medicine today becomes mere commonsense tomorrow . . .[15]

Yet I do not believe that we are ready to let Adolf Meyer fade quietly from the scene. We still have some lessons to learn from him. I am not sighing for the glories of yesteryear. We cannot turn back; psychoanalysis, social psychiatry, and other approaches have led us far beyond 1940; and I have touched upon the inadequacies of psychobiology as Meyer left it to us.

When we scrutinize the current scene, we must sometimes wonder how much has changed in the psychiatrists' comprehension of the nature of the problems of psychiatry. We find that just as when Meyer became pathologist at Kankakee, many psychiatrists are seeking the causes of mental disorders in following up the latest discoveries in neurochemistry, neurophysiology, and endocrinology. There is, of course, nothing wrong with studying these factors, and, indeed, a great need to do so. Trouble arises when they are still searching for "something else" that can be measured or analyzed chemically to explain experience and behavior; or insist that the study of the patient's life cannot be scientific; or when they seek to avoid the complexities that arise from consideration of problems of living by focusing on but a single element. What, then, has become of the concept of the psychobiological level of integration that had proved so useful?

We note that recently a prominent psychiatrist wrote a book in which he found it necessary to insist that mental disorders are not illnesses. What, then, has happened to Meyer's reaction patterns that we accepted years ago and which have been a hallmark of American psychiatry?

Too, when we consider psychoanalysis, which replaced psychobiology on the conductor's podium and brought such notable advances, we find that its leadership has faltered and now virtually halted. There have been few significant advances in recent years. To some extent psychoanalysis is paying the penalty for the premature systematizations about which Meyer complained. Theorists have been striving to overcome the early overemphasis on id psychology, to make a place for the conscious decision-making functions of the ego, and to include concerns with problems of adaptation to the social environment. It is, however, difficult to alter premises or concepts that have served as a foundation for the theoretic structure; and it is difficult to sort out the unessential ideas that were introduced to buttress faulty premises.

The problems do not derive so much from specific concepts that must be replaced as from difficulties in the basic orientation. Psychoanalysis has remained unusually firmly tied to the patterns of thought of the time and place of its origin. Some of its underlying assumptions are more suited to metaphysics than science, and others more attuned to a belief system. There is, of course, no room in science for loyalty to a theory or even to a person, but simply to the pursuit of truth wherever it may lead; nor is there room for the invocation of authority as proof of a concept's validity; nor for the search after truth through the exegesis of writings.

It is difficult for a psychiatric theory that still contains Lamarckian ideas to relate properly to the corpus of science as a whole; or one that uses a model of a closed energy system for an animal organism, or places in a central position an energy system that no other branch of biology recognizes and for which it has neither produced evidence nor a necessity for postulating. Too difficult to discuss with brevity are those ideas related to metaphysics that seek an ultimate truth, and which contain strong residues of a disembodied mind whose structure can be ascertained through the exercise of pure reason. As Alfred North Whitehead has pointed out, those principles that are on the fringe of consciousness, or which underlie our assumptions, may not seem to determine our thinking, but in fact, they play a major role in what we can let ourselves see, what commands our interest, and in the way we think about it.

Although we may not realize it, many of us are caught up in an inherent conflict between some of the unrecognized assumptions of psychoanalysis and our instrumental pluralistic approach to the remainder of science. It seems very likely that if we apply some of our instrumental, pragmatic ideas, much of the conflict can be eliminated. If only we ask, "Does it make a difference?" and "Can the query be answered by experience?" a way may be found out of preoccupations and controversies that are closer to scholastic matching of wits than a challenge of nature. Progress in science, let us remember, does not come from mental processes and observation alone but from placing questions through which we force nature to reveal her secrets.

The point I am trying to make is simply that Meyer, by introducing instrumental and pluralistic concepts into psychiatry, had provided psychiatry with a fundamental scientific orientation that fitted into the remainder of science and at the same time opened the way for the inclusion of data concerning human experience and biography in biological thinking. Somehow, in turning toward the many advantages offered by psychoanalysis, we have gone far toward losing this instrumental approach and the advantages it provided for ordering our investigations. Herein lies the source of many of our current theoretical confusions. Ideas are important— they are plans for action.

Adolf Meyer virtually identified himself with psychiatry. Its gains were his gains. He would gladly have his resting place in the foundations of modern psychiatry and have his ideas become forgotten, buried sources of new and more useful concepts. He was a man of wisdom and perspective. I have tried to indicate that we still have a need for conscious awareness of his basic contributions. In commemorating him, we can do much for ourselves and for psychiatry by recognizing and utilizing the heritage he left us.

REFERENCES

1. Beers, C. *A Mind That Found Itself,* revised ed. Garden City, NY: Doubleday and Co., 1948.

2. Bleuler, M. Early Swiss Sources of Adolf Meyer's Concepts, *Amer. J. Psychiat.,* *119*:193-196, 1962.

3. Dewey, J. *Experience and Nature.* Lasalle, IL: Open Court Publishing Co., 1925.

4. Dewey, J. *The Quest for Certainty.* New York: Minton, Balch and Co. (Putnam), 1929.

5. James. W. *The Will to Believe and Other Essays in Popular Philosophy.* New York: Longmans, Green and Co., 1897.

6. James. W. *Pragmatism: A New Name for Some Old Ways of Thinking.* New York: Longmans, Green and Co., 1907.

7. James, W. *Essays in Radical Empiricism.* New York: Longmans, Green and Co., 1912.

8. Katzenelbogen, S., ed. *Contributions Dedicated to Dr. Adolf Meyer by His Colleagues, Friends and Pupils.* Baltimore: Johns Hopkins Press, 1938.

9. Lidz, T. Book review of Collected Papers of Adolf Meyer, Vols. I and II, *Bull. Hist. Med.,* 28:94-97, 1954.

10. Lidz, T. *The Family and Human Adaptation.* New York: International Universities Press, 1963.

11. Lidz, T. "Adolf Meyer," in *International Encyclopedia of the Social Sciences*, in press.

12. Lief, A. *The Commonsense Psychiatry of Dr. Adolf Meyer.* New York: McGraw-Hill Book Co., 1948.

13. Meyer, A. "The Treatment of the Insane" (1894), in *Collected Papers*, vol. 2. Baltimore: Johns Hopkins Press, 1952.

14. Meyer. A. On the Observation of Abnormalities of Childhood, *Child Study Monthly*, *1*:1, 1895. Reprinted in Collected Papers, vol. 2. Baltimore: Johns Hopkins Press, 1952.

15. Meyer, A. The "Complaint" as the Center of Genetic-Dynamic and Nosological Thinking in Psychiatry, *New Eng. J. Med.*, *199*:360-370, 1928. Reprinted in Collected Papers, vol. 3. Baltimore: Johns Hopkins Press, 1952.

16. Meyer, A. British Influences in Psychiatry and Mental Hygiene, *J. Ment. Sci.*, *79*: 435-464, 1933. Reprinted in Collected Papers, vol. 3. Baltimore: Johns Hopkins Press, 1952.

17. Meyer, A. *Collected Papers*, 4 vols., E. Winters, ed. Baltimore: Johns Hopkins Press, 1952.

18. Meyer, A. *Psychobiology* (the 1932 Salmon Lectures), E. Winters and A. M. Bowers, eds. Springfield, IL: Charles C. Thomas, 1957.

19. Muller, S. F. *Amerikanische Philosophie.* Stuttgart: Fr. Fromanns Verlag, 1936.

20. Peirce, C. S. *Essays in the Philosophy of Science.* Philadelphia: Bobbs-Merrill Co., 1957.

21. Perry, R. B. *The Thought and Character of William James*, vol. 2. Boston: Little, Brown and Co., 1935.

22. Ratner, J. *Introduction: Intelligence in the Modern World: John Dewey's Philosophy.* New York: Modern Library, 1939.

23. Smith, J.E. *The Spirit of American Philosophy.* New York: Oxford University Press, 1963.

24. Smuts, J. C. *Holism and Evolution.* New York: Macmillan Co., 1926.

25. Zilboorg, G. & Henry, S. W. *A History of Medical Psychology.* New York: W. W. Norton and Co., 1941.

Habit

William James

ITS IMPORTANCE FOR PSYCHOLOGY

There remains a condition of general neural activity so important as to deserve a chapter by itself—I refer to the aptitude of the nerve-centres, especially of the hemispheres, for acquiring habits. *An acquired habit, from the physiological point of view, is nothing but a new pathway of discharge formed in the brain, by which certain incoming currents ever after tend to escape.* That is the thesis of this chapter; and we shall see in the later and more psychological chapters that such functions as the association of ideas, perception, memory, reasoning, the education of the will, etc., etc., can best be understood as results of the formation *de novo* of just such pathways of discharge.

Habit has a physical basis. The moment one tries to define what habit is, one is led to the fundamental properties of matter. The laws of Nature are nothing but the immutable habits which the different elementary sorts of matter follow in their actions and reactions upon each other. In the organic world, however, the habits are more variable than this. Even instincts vary from one individual to another of a kind; and are modified in the same individual, as we shall later see, to suit the exigencies of the case. On the principles of the atomistic philosophy the habits of an elementary particle of matter cannot change, because the particle is itself an unchangeable thing; but those of a compound mass of matter can change, because they are in the last instance due to the structure of the compound, and either outward forces or inward tensions can, from one hour to another, turn that structure into something different from what it was. That is, they can do so if the body be plastic enough to maintain its integrity, and be not disrupted when its structure yields. The change of structure here spoken of need not involve the outward shape; it

This article is reprinted from *Psychology, Briefer Course,* Chapter 10, NY: Holt, 1892.
    The material in this section represents basic elements in James's psychology and provides the background for an understanding of his philosophical development.

may be invisible and molecular, as when a bar of iron becomes magnetic or crystalline through the action of certain outward causes, or india-rubber becomes friable, or plaster "sets." All these changes are rather slow; the material in question opposes a certain resistance to the modifying cause, which it takes time to overcome, but the gradual yielding whereof often saves the material from being disintegrated altogether. When the structure has yielded, the same inertia becomes a condition of its comparative permanence in the new form, and of the new habits the body then manifests. *Plasticity,* then, in the wide sense of the word, means the possession of a structure weak enough to yield to an influence, but strong enough not to yield all at once. Each relatively stable phase of equilibrium in such a structure is marked by what we may call a new set of habits. Organic matter, especially nervous tissue, seems endowed with a very extraordinary degree of plasticity of this sort; so that we may without hesitation lay down as our first proposition the following: that *the phenomena of habit in living beings are due to the plasticity of the organic materials of which their bodies are composed.*

The philosophy of habit is thus, in the first instance, a chapter in physics rather than physiology or psychology. That it is at bottom a physical principle is admitted by all good recent writers on the subject. They call attention to analogues of acquired habits exhibited by dead matter. Thus, M. Léon Dumont writes:

> Every one knows how a garment, after having been worn a certain time, clings to the shape of the body better than when it was new; there has been a change in the tissue, and this change is a new habit of cohesion. A lock works better after being used some time: at the outset more force was required to overcome certain roughness in the mechanism. The overcoming of their resistance is a phenomenon of habituation. It costs less trouble to fold a paper when it has been folded already; . . . and just so in the nervous system the impressions of outer objects fashion for themselves more and more appropriate paths, and these vital phenomena recur under similar excitements from without, when they have been interrupted a certain time.

Not in the nervous system alone. A scar anywhere is a *locus minoris resistentiæ,* more liable to be abraded, inflamed, to suffer pain and cold, than are the neighboring parts. A sprained ankle, a dislocated arm, are in danger of being sprained or dislocated again;

joints that have once been attacked by rheumatism or gout, mucous membranes that have been the seat of catarrh, are with each fresh recurrence more prone to a relapse, until often the morbid state chronically substitutes itself for the sound one. And in the nervous system itself it is well known how many so-called functional diseases seem to keep themselves going simply because they happen to have once begun; and how the forcible cutting short by medicine of a few attacks is often sufficient to enable the physiological forces to get possession of the field again, and to bring the organs back to functions of health. Epilepsies, neuralgias, convulsive affections of various sorts, insomnias, are so many cases in point. And, to take what are more obviously habits, the success with which a "weaning" treatment can often be applied to the victims of unhealthy indulgence of passion, or of mere complaining or irascible disposition, shows us how much the morbid manifestations themselves were due to the mere inertia of the nervous organs, when once launched on a false career.

Habits are due to pathways through the nerve-centres. If habits are due to the plasticity of materials to outward agents, we can immediately see to what outward influences, if to any, the brain-matter is plastic. Not to mechanical pressures, not to thermal changes, not to any of the forces to which all the other organs of our body are exposed; for, as we [previously] saw, Nature has so blanketed and wrapped the brain about that the only impressions that can be made upon it are through the blood, on the one hand, and the sensory nerve-roots on the other; and it is to the infinitely attenuated currents that pour in through these latter channels that the hemispherical cortex shows itself to be so peculiarly susceptible. The currents, once in, must find a way out. In getting out they leave their traces in the paths which they take. The only thing they *can* do, in short, is to deepen old paths or to make new ones; and the whole plasticity on the brain sums itself up in two words when we call it an organ in which currents pouring in from the sense-organs make with extreme facility paths which do not easily disappear. For, of course, a simple habit, like every other nervous event—the habit of snuffling, for example, or of putting one's hands into one's pockets, or of biting one's nails—is, mechanically, nothing but a reflex discharge; and its anatomical substratum must be a path in the system. The most complex habits, as we shall presently see more fully, are, from the same point of view, nothing but *concatenated* discharges in the nerve-centres, due to the presence there of systems of reflex paths, so organized as to wake each other up successively—the impression produced by one muscular contraction serving as a stimulus to provoke the next, until a final impression inhibits the process and closes the chain.

It must be noticed that the growth of structural modification in living matter may be more rapid than in any lifeless mass, because the incessant nutritive renovation of which the living matter is the seat tends often to corroborate and fix the impressed modification, rather than to counteract it by renewing the original constitution of the tissue that has been impressed. Thus, we notice after exercising our muscles or our brain in a new way, that we can do so no longer at that time; but after a day or two of rest, when we resume the discipline, our increase in skill not seldom surprises us. I have often noticed this in learning a tune; and it has led a German author to say that we learn to swim during the winter, and to skate during the summer.

PRACTICAL EFFECTS OF HABIT

First, habit simplifies our movements, makes them accurate, and diminishes fatigue.

Man is born with a tendency to do more things than he has ready-made arrangements for in his nerve-centres. Most of the performances of other animals are automatic. But in him the number of them is so enormous that most of them must be in the fruit of painful study. If practice did not make perfect, nor habit economize the expense of nervous and muscular energy, he would be in a sorry plight. As Dr. Maudsley says:*

> If an act became easier after being done several times, if the careful direction of consciousness were necessary to its accomplishment on each occasion, it is evident that the whole activity of a lifetime might be confined to one or two deeds—that no progress could take place in development. A man might be occupied all day in dressing and undressing himself; the attitude of his body would absorb all his attention and energy; the washing of his hands or the fastening of a button would be as difficult to him on each occasion as to the child on its first trial;

---

*The Physiology of Mind, p. 155.

and he would, furthermore, be completely exhausted by his exertions. Think of the pains necessary to teach a child to stand, of the many efforts which it must make, and of the ease with which it at last stands, unconscious of any effort. For while secondarily-automatic acts are accomplished with comparatively little weariness—in this regard approaching the organic movements, or the original reflex movements—the conscious effort of the will soon produces exhaustion. A spinal cord without . . . memory would simply be an idiotic spinal cord. . . . It is impossible for an individual to realize how much he owes to its automatic agency until disease has impaired its functions.

Secondly, *habit diminishes the conscious attention with which our acts are performed.*

One may state this abstractly thus: If an act require for its execution a chain, *A, B, C, D, E, F, G,* etc., of successive nervous events, then in the first performances of the action the conscious will must choose each of these events from a number of wrong alternatives that tend to present themselves; but habit soon brings it about that each event calls up its own appropriate successor without any alternative offering itself, and without any reference to the conscious will, until at last the whole chain, *A, B, C, D, E, F, G,* rattles itself off as soon as *A* occurs, just as if *A* and the rest of the chain were fused into a continuous stream. Whilst we are learning to walk, to ride, to swim, skate, fence, write, play, or sing. we interrupt ourselves at every step by unnecessary movements and false notes. When we are proficients, on the contrary, the results follow not only with the very minimum of muscular action requisite to bring them forth, but they follow from a single instantaneous "cue." The marksman sees the bird, and, before he knows it, he has aimed and shot. A gleam in his adversary's eye, a momentary pressure from his rapier, and the fencer finds that he has instantly made the right parry and return. A glance at the musical hieroglyphics, and the pianist's fingers have rippled through a shower of notes. And not only is it the right thing at the right time that we thus involuntarily do, but the wrong thing also, if it be an habitual thing. Who is there that has never wound up his watch on taking off his waistcoat in the daytime, or taken his latch-key out on arriving at the doorstep of a friend? Persons in going to their bedroom to dress for dinner have been known to take off one garment after another and finally to get into bed, merely because that was the habitual issue of the first few movements when performed at a later hour. We all have a definite routine manner of performing certain daily offices connected with the toilet, with the opening and shutting of familiar cupboards, and the like. But our higher thought-centres know hardly anything about the matter. Few men can tell off-hand which sock, shoe, or trousers-leg they put on first. They must first mentally rehearse the act; and even that is often insufficient—the act must be *performed.* So of the questions, Which valve of the shutters opens first? Which way does my door swing? etc. I cannot *tell* the answer; yet my *hand* never makes a mistake. No one can *describe* the order in which he brushes his hair or teeth; yet it is likely that the order is a pretty fixed one in all of us.

These results may be expressed as follows.

In action grown habitual, what instigates each new muscular contraction to take place in its appointed order is not a thought or a perception, but the *sensation occasioned by the muscular contraction just finished.* A strictly voluntary act has to be guided by idea, perception, and volition, throughout its whole course. In habitual action, mere sensation is a sufficient guide, and the upper regions of brain and mind are set comparatively free. A diagram will make the matter clear.

Let *A, B, C, D, E, F, G* represent an habitual chain of muscular contractions, and let *a, b, c, d, e, f* stand for the several sensations which these contractions excite in us when they are successively performed. Such sensations will usually be in the parts moved, but they may also be effects of the movement upon the eye or the ear. Through them, and through them alone, we are made aware whether or not the contraction has occurred. When the series, *A, B, C, D, E, F, G* is being learned, each of these sensations becomes the object of a separate act of attention by the mind. We test each movement intellectually, to see if it have been rightly performed, before advancing to the next. We hesitate, compare, choose, revoke, reject, etc.; and the order by which the next movement is discharged is an express order from the ideational centres after this deliberation has been gone through.

In habitual action, on the contrary, the only impulse which the intellectual centres need send down is that which carries the command to *start.* This is represented in the diagram by *V;* it may be a thought of the first movement or of the last result, or a mere perception of

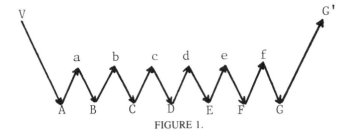
FIGURE 1.

some of the habitual conditions of the chain, the presence, e.g., of the keyboard near the hand. In the present example, no sooner has this conscious thought or volition instigated movement *A,* than *A,* through the sensation *a* of its own occurrence, awakens *B* reflexly; *B* then excites *C* through *b,* and so on till the chain is ended, when the intellect generally takes cognizance of the final result. The intellectual perception at the end is indicated in the diagram by the sensible effect of the movement *G* being represented at *G',* in the ideational centres above the merely sensational line. The sensational impressions, *a, b, c, d, e, f,* are all supposed to have their seat below the ideational level.

Habits depend on sensations not attended to. We have called *a, b, c, d, e, f,* by the name of "sensations." If sensations, they are sensations to which we are usually inattentive; but that they are more than unconscious nerve-currents seems certain, for they catch our attention if they go wrong. Schneider's account of these sensations deserves to be quoted. In the act of walking, he says, "even when our attention is entirely absorbed elsewhere, it is doubtful whether we could preserve equilibrium if no sensation of our body's attitude were there, and doubtful whether we should advance our leg if we had no sensation of its movement as executed, and not even a minimal feeling of impulse to set it down. Knitting appears altogether mechanical, and the knitter keeps up her knitting even while she reads or is engaged in lively talk. But if we ask her how this is possible, she will hardly reply that the knitting goes on of itself. She will rather say that she has a feeling of it, that she feels in her hands that she knits and how she must knit, and that therefore the movements of knitting are called forth and regulated by the sensations associated therewithal, even when the attention is called away. . . ." Again: "When a pupil begins to play on the violin, to keep him from raising his right elbow in playing a book is placed under his right armpit, which he is ordered to hold fast by keeping the upper arm tight against his body. The muscular feelings, and feelings of contact connected with the book, provoke an impulse to press it tight. But often it happens that the beginner, whose attention gets absorbed in the production of the notes, lets drop the book. Later, however, this never happens; the faintest sensations of contact suffice to awaken the impulse to keep it in its place, and the attention may be wholly absorbed by the notes and the fingering with the left hand. *The simultaneous combination of movements is thus in the first instance conditioned by the facility with which in us, alongside of intellectual processes, processes of inattentive feeling may still go on.*''

ETHICAL AND PEDAGOGICAL IMPORTANCE OF THE PRINCIPLE OF HABIT

''Habit a second nature! Habit is ten times nature,'' the Duke of Wellington is said to have exclaimed; and the degree to which this is true no one probably can appreciate as well as one who is a veteran soldier himself. The daily drill and the years of discipline end by fashioning a man completely over again, as to most of the possibilities of his conduct.

''There is a story,'' says Prof. Huxley, ''which is credible enough, though it may not be true, of a practical joker who, seeing a discharged veteran carrying home his dinner, suddenly called out, 'Attention!' whereupon the man instantly brought his hands down, and lost his mutton and potatoes in the gutter. The drill had been thorough, and its effects had become embodied in the man's nervous structure.''

Riderless cavalry horses, at many a battle, have been seen to come together and go through their customary evolutions at the sound of the bugle-call. Most domestic beasts seem machines almost pure and simple, undoubtingly, unhesitatingly doing from minute to minute the duties they have been taught, and giving no sign that the possibility of an alternative ever suggests itself to their mind. Men grown old in prison have asked to be readmitted after being once set free. In a railroad accident a menagerie-tiger, whose cage had broken open, is said to have emerged, but presently crept back again, as if too much bewildered by his new responsibilities, so that he was without difficulty secured.

Habit is thus the enormous fly-wheel of society, its most precious conservative agent. It alone is what keeps us all within the bounds of ordinance, and saves the children of fortune from the envious uprisings of the poor. It alone prevents the hardest and most repulsive walks of life from being deserted by those brought up to tread therein. It keeps the fisherman and the deck-hand at sea through the winter; it holds the miner in his darkness, and nails the countryman to his log-cabin and his lonely farm through all the months of snow; it protects us from invasion by the natives of the desert and the frozen zone. It dooms us all to fight out the battle of life upon the lines of our nurture or our early choice, and to make the best of a pursuit that disagrees, because there is no other for which we are fitted, and it is too late to begin again. It keeps different social strata from mixing. Already at the age of twenty-five you see the professional mannerism settling down on the young commercial traveller, on the young doctor, on the young minister, on the young counsellor-at-law. You see the little lines of cleavage running through the character, the tricks of thought, the prejudices, the ways of the "shop," in a word, from which the man can by-and-by no more escape than his coat-sleeve can suddenly fall into a new set of folds. On the whole, it is best he should not escape. It is well for the world that in most of us, by the age of thirty, the character has set like plaster, and will never soften again.

If the period between twenty and thirty is the critical one in the formation of intellectual and professional habits, the period below twenty is more important still for the fixing of *personal* habits, properly so called, such as vocalization and pronunciation, gesture, motion, and address. Hardly ever is a language learned after twenty spoken without a foreign accent; hardly ever can a youth transferred to the society of his betters unlearn the nasality and other vices of speech bred in him by the associations of his growing years. Hardly ever, indeed, no matter how much money there be in his pocket, can he even learn to *dress* like a gentleman-born. The merchants offer their wares as eagerly to him as to the veriest "swell," but he simply *cannot* buy the right things. An invisible law, as strong as gravitation, keeps him within his orbit, arrayed this year as he was the last; and how his better-clad acquaintances contrive to get the things they wear will be for him a mystery till his dying day.

The great thing, then, in all education, is to *make our nervous system our ally instead of our enemy.* It is to fund and capitalize our acquisitions, and live at ease upon the interest of the fund. *For this we must make automatic and habitual, as early as possible, as many useful actions as we can,* and guard against the growing into ways that are likely to be disadvantageous to us, as we should guard against the plague. The more of the details of our daily life we can hand over to the effortless custody of automatism, the more our higher powers of mind will be set free for their own proper work. There is no more miserable human being than one in whom nothing is habitual but indecision, and for whom the lighting of every cigar, the drinking of every cup, the time of rising and going to bed every day, and the beginning of every bit of work, are subjects of express volitional deliberation. Full half the time of such a man goes to the deciding, or regretting, of matters which ought to be so ingrained in him as practically not to exist for his consciousness at all. If there be such daily duties not yet ingrained in any one of my readers, let him begin this very hour to set the matter right.

In Professor Bain's chapter on ''The Moral Habits'' there are some admirable practical remarks laid down. Two great maxims emerge from his treatment. The first is that in the acquisition of a new habit, or the leaving off of an old one, we must take care to *launch ourselves with as strong and decided an initiative as possible.* Accumulate all the possible circumstances which shall re-enforce the right motives; put yourself assiduously in conditions that encourage the new way; make engagements incompatible with the old; take a public pledge, if the case allows; in short, envelop your resolution with every aid you know. This will give your new beginning such a momentum that the temptation to break down will not occur as soon as it otherwise might; and every day during which a break-down is postponed adds to the chances of its not occurring at all.

The second maxim is: *Never suffer an exception to occur till the new habit is securely rooted in your life.* Each lapse is like the letting fall of a ball of string which one is carefully winding up; a single slip undoes more than a great many turns will wind again. *Continuity* of training is the great means of making the nervous system act infallibly right. As Professor Bain says:

> The peculiarity of the moral habits, contradistinguishing them from the intellectual acquisitions, is the presence of two hostile powers, one to be gradually raised into the ascendant over the other. It is necessary, above all things, in such a situation, never to lose a battle. Every gain on the wrong side undoes the effect of many conquests on the right. The essential precau-

tion, therefore, is so to regulate the two opposing powers that the one may have a series of uninterrupted successes, until repetition has fortified it to such a degree as to enable it to cope with the opposition, under any circumstances. This is the theoretically best career of mental progress.

The need of securing success at the *outset* is imperative. Failure at first is apt to damp the energy of all future attempts, whereas past experiences of success nerve one to future vigor. Goethe says to a man who consulted him about an enterprise but mistrusted his own powers: "Ach! you need only blow on your hands!" And the remark illustrates the effect on Goethe's spirits of his own habitually successful career.

The question of "tapering-off," in abandoning such habits as drink and opium-indulgence comes in here, and is a question about which experts differ within certain limits, and in regard to what may be best for an individual case. In the main, however, all expert opinion would agree that abrupt acquisition of the new habit is the best way, *if there be a real possibility of carrying it out.* We must be careful not to give the will so stiff a task as to insure its defeat at the very outset; but, *provided one can stand it,* a sharp period of suffering, and then a free time, is the best thing to aim at, whether in giving up a habit like that of opium, or in simply changing one's hours of rising or of work. It is surprising how soon a desire will die of inanition if it be *never* fed.

> One must first learn, unmoved, looking neither to the right nor left, to walk firmly on the strait and narrow path, before one can begin "to make one's self over again." He who every day makes a fresh resolve is like one who, arriving at the edge of the ditch he is to leap, forever stops and returns for a fresh run. Without *unbroken* advance there is no such thing as *accumulation* of the ethical forces possible, and to make this possible, and to exercise us and habituate us in it, is the sovereign blessing of regular work.*

A third maxim may be added to the preceding pair: *Seize the very first possible opportunity to act on every resolution you make, and on every emotional prompting you may experience in the direction of*

---

*J. Bahnsen: *Beitrage zu Charakterologie* (1867), vol. I, p. 209.

the habits you aspire to gain. It is not in the moment of their forming, but in the moment of their producing *motor effects,* that
resolves and aspirations communicate the new "set" to the brain.
As the author last quoted remarks:

> The actual presence of the practical opportunity alone fur-
> nishes the fulcrum upon which the lever can rest, by means of
> which the moral will may multiply its strength, and raise itself
> aloft. He who has no solid ground to press against will never
> get beyond the stage of empty gesture-making.

No matter how full a reservoir of *maxims* one may possess, and
no matter how good one's *sentiments* may be, if one have not taken
advantage of every concrete opportunity to *act,* one's character may
remain entirely unaffected for the better. With mere good intentions, hell is proverbially paved. And this is an obvious consequence
of the principles we have laid down. A "character," as J. S. Mill
says, "is a completely fashioned will"; and a will, in the sense in
which he means it, is an aggregate of tendencies to act in a firm and
prompt and definite way upon all the principal emergencies of life.
A tendency to act only becomes effectively ingrained in us in proportion to the uninterrupted frequency with which the actions actually occur, and the brain "grows" to their use. When a resolve or a
fine glow of feeling is allowed to evaporate without bearing practical fruit it is worse than a chance lost; it works so as positively to
hinder future resolutions and emotions from taking the normal path
of discharge. There is no more contemptible type of human character than that of the nerveless sentimentalist and dreamer, who
spends his life in a weltering sea of sensibility and emotion, but who
never does a manly concrete deed. Rousseau, inflaming all the
mothers of France, by his eloquence, to follow Nature and nurse
their babies themselves, while he sends his own children to the
foundling hospital, is the classical example of what I mean. But
every one of us in his measure, whenever, after glowing for an abstractly formulated Good, he practically ignores some actual case,
among the squalid "other particulars" of which that same Good
lurks disguised, treads straight on Rousseau's path. All Goods are
disguised by the vulgarity of their concomitants, in this work-a-day
world; but woe to him who can only recognize them when he thinks
them in their pure and abstract form! The habit of excessive novel-
reading and theatre-going will produce true monsters in this line.

The weeping of the Russian lady over the fictitious personages in the play, while her coachman is freezing to death on his seat outside, is the sort of thing that everywhere happens on a less glaring scale. Even the habit of excessive indulgence in music, for those who are neither performers themselves nor musically gifted enough to take it in a purely intellectual way, has probably a relaxing effect upon character. One becomes filled with emotions which habitually pass without prompting to any deed, and so the inertly sentimental condition is kept up. The remedy would be, never to suffer one's self to have an emotion at a concert, without expressing it afterward in *some* active way. Let the expression be the least thing in the world—speaking genially to one's grandmother, or giving up one's seat in horse-car, if nothing more heroic offers—but let it not fail to take place.

Adolf Meyer:
Contributions to the Conceptual
Foundation of Occupational Therapy

Karen Diasio Serrett
Stacy Newbury
Alice Tabacco
Janis Trimble

Adolf Meyer was a prominent figure in American psychiatry during the late 1800s and early 1900s. Originally a neuropathologist, his interests began to shift "to the living" (Lief, 1948). He began interviewing patients and found that often their life stories bore an explanation for their illness. He developed the fundamentals of his theory which he termed Psychobiology. Meyer stated that "Psychobiology starts not from a mind and body or from elements, but from the fact that we deal with biologically organized units and groups and their functioning" (Lief, 1948).

In October of 1921, he presented his fundamental thinking on occupational therapy at the Fifth Annual Meeting of the National Society for the Promotion of Occupational Therapy in his classic paper, "Philosophy of Occupation Therapy." Most occupational therapists are quite familiar with this work, but have not had access to other memorable statements from Meyer that may be of equal interest for their articulation of the founding beliefs, philosophies, and principles of occupational therapy. This summary of statements and quotes will hopefully give occupational therapists and other professionals a deeper appreciation for the startling relevance of his thinking for the emerging Systems Age.

PSYCHOBIOLOGICAL THEORY

"We have come to speak of mind or soul as the person's *nature* or *function, not* as if we meant something detached; . . . We sense a *complete person* with flesh and blood, a product of growth, cerebrally and functionally integrated, an active entity, exhibiting what was spoken of by Charles Mercier even in the nineties as *conduct* and later by William McDougall and others as *behavior.*''

1933. British influences in psychiatry and mental hygiene. *Journal of Mental Science,* 79, 435.

''Since the other elements which are apt to figure in our presentations of etiology, nosology, and pathology are much more hazy, it is more satisfactory to come out frankly with a statement that we wish to take distinctions of various types of habit disorganization, to study the working of the various sets of activities and habits of the patient, determine their relative values by accurate observation coming up to the mark of the experiment and shaping our therapeutic measures in accord with these principles.''

1912. Studies in psychiatry. *Nervous and Mental Disease Monograph Series,* No. 9, 1, 95.

''In speaking of 'mental integrations' I imply the whole of our attitudes and activities, including the respiratory and vasomotor and circulatory and cerebral activity involved, and also the situation in which the reaction takes place as a process of adjustment. The 'integrations of the nervous system' would thus form an essential link in the broader 'integration of the personality.' ''

1912. Paper read to joint session of the American Psychological Association and the Southern Society for Philosophy and Psychology. *Journal of the American Medical Association,* 58, 911.

''I urge the student to trace the plain life history of a person and to record it on what I call the life chart; the result is a record of a smooth or broken life curve of each one of the main organs and functions, and, in addition, a record of the main events of the life of the whole bundle of organs, that is, 'the individual as a whole,' and of the facts which determined and constituted his behavior.''

1912-1913. Presidential Address, American Psychopathological Association. *Journal of Abnormal Psychology,* 1, 313.

''The field of human total-function or psychobiology is probably the one domain of science that presents not so much a mass of new information as primarily training in using what everybody knows. I regard the course as one of organizing the best critical common-sense in a form usable in record keeping and in serious work with patients. It is not merely a preparation for psychiatry; it means to serve all our dealings with human beings.''

> 1935. Scope and teaching of psychobiology in the first year of medical school. *Journal of the Association of American Medical Colleges,* 10, 93, 365.

''Psychobiology as thus conceived forms clearly and simply the missing chapter of ordinary physiology and pathology, the chapter dealing with functions of the total person and not merely of detachable parts.''

> 1915. Address to the American Medical Association. *Journal of the American Medical Association,* 65, 860.

ON OCCUPATION

''We have learned to meet on concrete ground the real essence of mind and soul—the plain and intelligible human activities and relations to self and others.''

> 1921. Address at the celebration of the 100th anniversary of Bloomingdale Hospital, White Plains, N.Y.

Occupation is, with good right, called the most essential side of hygienic treatment of most insane patients.

> 1893. Paper to the Chicago Pathological Society.

''Our concern is with the events or 'doings,' not with the being or final essence, and therein lies the great difference between the old frame of thought and the modern one. . . . The concept of activity is one of the most useful and harmless formulas of expressions of events, emphasizing the importance of the role played by the 'subject.' ''

> 1907. Misconceptions at the bottom of ''hopelessness of all psychology.'' *Psychological Bulletin,* 4, 170.

''Psychotherapy is regulation of action and only complete when action is reached. This is why we all use it in the form of occupation or rest, where it is an efficient and controllable form of regulation. This is why we teach patients to actually take different attitudes to things. Habit training is the backbone of psychotherapy. . . .''

> 1908. The role of mental factors in psychiatry. *American Journal of Insanity,* 65, 39.

"There would be far more happiness and real success in mental hygiene if more people would realize that at every step, every person can do *something* well and take a satisfaction in doing it, and that this satisfaction in something *done* is to be valued as ten times greater than the satisfaction taken in mere thought or imagination, however lofty.

"It must be remembered that thought at its very best is only a link in a chain of events leading up to some achievement. Its real and lasting fulfillment is found only in action. Janet has constructed an interesting hierarchy of mental functions. His study of psychasthenia brings him to the conviction that *complete action* is the most difficult and highest function. I am tempted to add that completed action is the first essential for rest and for beginning something new.

"To sum up, I should urge that we spread among teachers and pupils a realization of the fact that knowledge must be a knowledge *ready for doing* things. Even in cultivating the instincts of play and pleasure we must aim to make as attractive as possible those games and diversions which require decision and action, and carry with them a prompt demand for correction of mistakes and reward for achievement: actual play with others and for others, and not the play of mere rumination. We further must aim to find levels of activity with moderate demands and well within the limitations of even the less brilliant or less vigorous children and yet giving full enough satisfaction to remain attractive and truly stimulating."

> 1908. What do histories of cases of insanity teach us concerning preventive mental hygiene during the years of school life? Read to the American School Hygiene Association, April, 1908. *Psychological Clinic,* 2, 89.

"Prophylaxis is the climax and fulfillment of our endeavor in after-care work. . . . As a matter of fact, I have already felt that the term 'after-care' as it was established in England, that is to say, one or two months' care for people who are discharged and need a boarding place or something of that nature, but it consists of finding occupation for patients who are leaving the institution and trying to live again in the community, and helping to make their reentrance into the community easy and safe against relapses.''

1909. Discussion of After-Care Committee Meeting, Willard State Hospital. *State Hospitals Bulletin,* 1, 631.

''A little less worry over the child and a bit more concern about the world we make for the child to live in; an inclusion of the child in a life of which the aim is not merely to earn money so as to become independent of the job; more love for wholehearted, creative work and progress that will make possible what we all can share in. . . .''

1915. Address to the American Medical Association. *Journal of the American Medical Association,* 65, 860.

ANTICIPATING SYSTEMS AGE THINKING

'' 'My struggle in this country,' [Meyer] told me, 'has been with a false conception of science.' Mistaken science, using test tube and microscope as its symbols, talked about and claimed to know more and more about less and less such as the alleged importance of cell nuclei. 'Psychiatry has to be found in the function and the life of the people.' '' (Lief, 1948, p. vii).

''One of the first things that has proved of value in this direction has been the abandonment of fussing over the supposed *elements* of psychology and the attempts to explain chains of events out of such elements. It proved to be much more satisfactory to speak in terms of situation, reaction, and final adjustment and to describe all the facts of interaction according to their weight without excessive scruples over the systematization of what will be the last thing to reach a stage. . . . It is better to use the broad concepts of instincts, habits, interests, and specific experiences and capacities, than the concepts of structural analysis at the present stage of our biological knowledge.''

1908. The problem of mental reaction-types, mental causes and diseases. *Psychological Bulletin,* 5, 245.

''To try and explain a hysterical fit or delusion system out of hypothetical cell alterations which we cannot reach or prove is at the present stage of histophysiology a gratuitous performance. To realize that such a reaction is a *faulty response or substitution of an insufficient or protective or evasive or mutilated attempt at adjustment* opens ways of inquiry in the direction of modifiable determining factors and all of a sudden we find ourselves in a live field, in harmony with our instincts of action, of prevention, of modification, and of an understanding, doing justice to a desire for directness instead of neurologizing tautology.''

> 1912. The relationship of hysteria, psychasthenia, and dementia praecox. *Nervous and Mental Disease Monograph Series,* No. 9, 1, 55.

''For all I can see, the main obstacle to a wider acceptance of a functional theory in terms of habit and complex conflicts and definite responses thereto it is on the one hand the habitual or intentional lack of the necessary penetration into the life of the patient and family, and on the other hand the readiness of the physician to turn to set interpretations and to reiterate authoritative statements with a certain pedagogical self-sufficiency.''

> 1910. Lecture at the celebration of the 25th anniversary of Clark University, Worcester, Mass. American Journal of Psychology, 21, 385.

''While the elementary sciences pride themselves on getting along with elements which stand by themselves, embodying as it were with fatal necessity all the effects into which they can be led, the living organism, owing to its complexity, baffles the demand for regularity in many points. Hence the temptation to fall into the mistake in which men like Loeb get involved when they believe that only a rigid mechanistic conception of nature can eliminate mysticism, and that any recognition of conditioned reactions and any temporary acceptance of a measure of factors in terms of the effect produced in the completion of a known process, . . . the entire logical formula of seeing parts in the light of a whole is to be replaced by, however hypothetical, constructs of elementary units, . . . is at least to be discredited. I should on the contrary, urge that the training in physiology, put much more emphasis on the definition of the conditions under which ends are attained.''

> 1912-1913. Presidential address, American Psychopathological Association. *Journal of Abnormal Psychology,* 7, 313.

REFERENCES

Lief, A. *The Commonsense Psychiatry of Adolf Meyer.* NY: McGraw-Hill, 1948.

Historical and Philosophical Bases of Psychobiology

Wendell Muncie

When the American Psychological Association in 1911 discussed the incorporation in the medical curricula of this country of some elementary facts concerning normal psychology, a momentous step in American medical education was instituted. Previously medical schools were graduating students trained in anatomy, physiology, and pathology, and with more or less consideration of abnormal behavior but with no training in observation and evaluation of normal behavior. Yet this was obviously a most urgent need, for whether or not the student would ever turn to the field of human behavior for his life's work, he must perforce deal with it in its manifold variations from the very moment of his first contact with his first patient. The action of the Association was the beginning therefore of a long deferred step toward a study of the whole of man, not only of parts.

Having taken that step, the next question was, What to teach? And at this point the good intentions of the Association were in danger of being wrecked through the fact that "psychology" was a Babel of tongues, each proclaiming with too much insistence its just and sole right to use the name: introspection psychology, motor psychology, and so on. On that occasion (1912) Adolf Meyer[1] presented a plan of teaching which offered a promise of positive assistance to the student. This plan began with the entirely practical suggestion that since everyone is the possessor of a not inconsiderable experiential knowledge of man, this body of common observation was the thing to begin with, to be organized and trained. In other words, the study of psychology should start with what was known, rather than the overparticular and oversystematized material of some of the current systems. Second, the student was as far as possible asked to reduce the observations on human behavior to terms of *actual overt performances,* open to observation by anyone who cared to look, without,

This article is reprinted Chapter 1 from *Psychobiology and Psychiatry,* St. Louis: C.V. Moseby, 1939.

Muncie's medical textbook was widely used to teach Meyer's belief and principles.

however, disregarding the more implicit activity, the thoughts, memories, etc., but including them as economizing performances or pictorial or verbal forerunners to overt performance. Third, the observations should be made by the student on himself, because the student knew more of himself than of anyone else, and it seemed the best way to bring home to the student how it feels to have personal issues handled. Nevertheless the facts should be essentially the same as those which others would want to describe and note. Fourth, the student was to compare the data of himself with those of three other dissimilar students, to give some idea of the range of variation of the normal, and to avoid the sense of mere introspection.

Such a program, it was felt, would serve to awaken in the student early in his career an alertness to problems with which he must deal throughout his medical career, and complete the familiarization with the "normal" begun in the courses of anatomy and physiology. The program rests on relatively neutral territory, using the accepted standards of scientific work: observation, experimentation, and control as far as the nature of the material allows. It leaves the door open for special data resting on the use of special concepts and methods, only demanding that they be subjected to ordinary scientific tests of validity.

The course was begun at the Johns Hopkins Medical School in 1913-14 and has continued since with growing acceptance among the student body of a rightful place in the curriculum. Similar courses have been inaugurated elsewhere, so that today it appears as an obligatory course in a large number of medical schools.

Adolf Meyer called the course one of objective "psychobiology," clinching a place for the study of man as a person clearly within the general framework of biology, the prefix "psycho" serving to emphasize the devotion to the reactions of the unitary organism, mentally integrated through symbolization and with more or less consciousness, in contrast to the function of more or less detachable parts and organs. The two terms, symbolization and consciousness, perhaps need clarification.

Symbolization is the process by which time-bound experience is represented in terms of pictures or perceptions and words with meaning, capable through this of influencing present and future behavior beyond the consequences of the experience, which would immediately and inevitably result from mere physiological integration of the functioning parts. For example, the knee jerk in healthy people results inevitably from a brisk tap on the quadriceps tendon. This "reflex" reaction can be shown to result from certain physiological nervous integrations involving principally the abruptly stretched quadriceps tendon and the afferent nerves from, and the motor nerves to, the quadriceps muscles and their central connections. This is the commonly expected reaction. It has nothing to do with any intention or memory and is identical with what can be produced in a mere reflex preparation in the physiological laboratory. But if, in a "nervous" person, the knee jerks forward *before* the hammer touches the person, only one conclusion can be made: the patient has anticipated the entire reaction and jerked the knee. It is the difference between the "knee jerk" of physiology and "the person jerking the knee" of psychobiology. Such a performance must have resulted from previous experience with the test, coupled with certain personal emotional attitudes in relation to it, as an anticipation reaction, with the general tension and fear of the examination. It could no doubt be shown that in its intimate detail this response is differently constituted, probably with special muscle combinations, and as a response with some meaning and intention for the patient as a person.

This example illustrates the essential elements of full-fledged mentally integrated activity of the total organism:

1. It depends on sensation.
2. The sensation is perceived; and with the introduction of the term perception the organismal activity has already been admitted, for perception is the result of the fusing of simple sensation and the associational material from experience or fancy it calls forth.
3. Motor performance results, which carries with it the earmarks of a "personal" reaction, something like but different from the simply physiological reflex in that it has meaning, in terms of experience, i.e., a part of personal biography.

There are various types or degrees of symbolization:

1. Perception of sensation is the simplest sort, depending on the associative tools of memory, and capable of influencing future action through fancy, anticipation, etc.
2. Pictorial and auditory (and other special sense) memories, leading to a systematization as elementary thought or lan-

guage, written and oral, closely related still to concrete experience.

3. Abstract concept formation, as seen in the further development of language through extension and restriction (simile, metaphor, identification, analogy, etc.), in the concept of number and its systematization as mathematics, and in the development of logic and philosophy—all further removed from actual experience and using formal rules of assumptions.

All perception, memory, imagination, fancy, anticipation, language and mathematics, logic, and philosophy are exercises in symbolization, linguistically elaborated only in the human. It can be shown by studies in comparative anatomy that those functions develop hand in hand with the increasing importance of the cerebral hemispheres.

"Consciousness" needs some clarification. It may appear bold to define a term which defied the efforts of the psychologists of the last century to delimit. The trouble with those efforts was that consciousness was conceived of as a static entity, the essence of "mental being," to be described in terms of sensory perceptions, and their interpretation obtained through introspection. One was either conscious or not conscious, and, by extension, conscious became synonymous with the mental life or "mind," in contrast to the not-conscious or the "physical" or body. In other words, the older attempts failed through being based on the mind-body misconceptions.

Consciousness in psychobiology describes a modality of organismal action, varying in degree from sleeping and dreaming, to waking and clearness of thinking, etc. The conscious—not conscious contrast is replaced by a conception of more or less consciousness, implying in common parlance, degrees of awakeness and awareness of the personal activities, i.e., degrees of a specific "state of function" about as one speaks of "states of matter," solid, liquid, gaseous.

Such a conception of consciousness welcomes any reasonable suggestion as to the neural basis which makes such performance possible, as for example Dandy's experience[2] with the regular production of coma on ligation of the left anterior cerebral artery. Likewise there remains complete freedom, yes, a need, to determine the causes of the variations and range in conscious awareness. Some of the important factors making for reduced awareness are:

1. Developmental inadequacy in the sense that the breadth of grasp of experience increases from infancy to maturity and declines with old age.
2. Fatigue, ill health—again when sufficient to cause a lowering of general grasp.
3. Emotional factors, which suppress or prohibit the awareness of certain special issues.
4. Divided attention from simultaneously acting stimuli, especially when they are conflicting.

These factors will receive attention in later chapters dealing with abnormal performances.

Physicians treat people who suffer or are afflicted in one way or another. These few words summarize in its entirety the history and the present scope of medicine, as a science, an art, a profession. This book would be unnecessary if it were not for the special interpretation physicians themselves (and others) have in the past given to the two principal words, "people" and "suffer." According to this interpretation, "people" refers to the physical body or live organism, and "suffer" refers to the untoward events or afflictions which can happen to that body—of a tangible sort, to be grasped by observation and the special technical extensions in laboratory equipment. The medical student in his first days at school is confronted with the dead remains of a human being to dissect, and later with a body for autopsy; only later does he meet with a living being to examine by special methods. For the purposes of the training for which he is being prepared, it matters not at all what kind of person the dead man was, how he lived, loved, worked, suffered. Neither do these things count much with the living patient being percussed or otherwise explored for training purposes. When it comes, however, to assuming responsibility for the care of such a live being, personal factors always play some role and often the dominant one.

Any attitude which excludes from the scientific study of man all those functions distinctively and uniquely human is the direct expression of the doctrine of dualism. First explicitly stated by the French philosopher Descartes, the doctrine holds that "body" and "mind" are two absolutely independent substances; the former capable of scientific observation since it possesses the quality of extension; the latter defying scientific method. It is true he sought some sort of harmony between these two principles by means of the pineal gland, and so perhaps foreshadowed the more modern efforts of psychophysical parallelism. The net result of his effort was to confine medical scientific study to the "physical," anatomical, and physiological, whereas the study of the mental functions fell into the hands of the philosophers, and notably the theologians.

The Cartesian doctrine doubtless was in part the result of the social pressure of the time. The exclusion of the study of the human from a proper science is all the more notable since ancient Greek philosophy had recognized its right to a place in science. Aristotle distinguished between the living and the nonliving worlds. He further saw clearly the proper relations and distinctions among (1) the feeding soul (anima vegetativa), (2) the perceptive soul (anima sensitiva), and (3) the thinking soul (anima cogitativa), characterizing thereby three levels of functions distinctive respectively of plants, of animals, and of man. Aristotle therefore saw natural science divided into discrete heterogeneous fields, determined by both *form* and *matter* (or quality and quantity). He fathered a "vitalistic" philosophy commonly held by biologists.

Descartes, however, had the beginnings of authority in support of his dualistic views in the neoplatonic school which taught the homogeneity of all natural sciences reducible logically to a study of quantity, i.e., mechanics. He was the father of the mechanistic philosophy, most popular among the physicists. Modern psychology began its effort at independence from the guardianship of philosophy and theology probably through the boldness of spirit inspired by the revolutionary liberalism of the early eighteenth century. Harassed by the Cartesian dogma, it began timidly with the study of the data of introspection, to which a certain glamour was added by the use of quantitative method. By analogy with the atomistic chemistry of the time, the distinctively human performances, especially the sense perceptions, and the intellectual assets of memory, retention, associative capacity, etc., were reduced to elements. Complex behavior was explained by building with these elements.

Useful as all this was, it ignored an obvious feature of human beings: that man is known largely by what he does and says. Interpreting activity or behavior in a very narrow mechanistic sense, a group of psychologists explored this territory, treating man in essence as a reflex machine, his motor doings being the inevitable result of sensory influences brought to bear on him. Then arose the "behaviorist" group and the conditioned reflex ideology.

Both the introspection-associationist and the behaviorist-conditioned reflex movements were bound to flourish and to wither early because they were rooted in an inadequate and logically untenable philosophy: that of Descartes and Plato. Both soon arrived at the point where universal common sense could no longer follow.

There is a clear need for a philosophy and a science of man which will include all we can know of chemistry, physics, anatomy, biology, *and* those things peculiarly human—and not shared by other natural beings—commonly called mental things, or simply "mind." Aristotle had offered on logical grounds and backed with keen observation a view of natural phenomena which met this problem in its broad implications. It remained for the modern conceptions of developmental evolution and of functional integration to bolster this view. This modern view was stated by Adolf Meyer. The cardinal points are:

1. There exists a relative discontinuity in the sciences based in all likelihood on (a) essential qualitative differences in the subject matter and (b) on limitations in methods of study. For example, "animate" and "inanimate" serve a very useful descriptive purpose for all practical purposes. That they cannot be taken to describe unalterably opposed categories of phenomena, with all the prejudicial distinctions likely to arise from them, must be conceded in light of the discovery by Friedrich Wohler in 1828 that the "organic" urea could be produced synthetically in the laboratory; and of the recent achievement of Professor Wendell M. Stanley[3] in changing the tobacco mosaic virus to the "inanimate" from the "animate" form and vice versa. The numerous elementary isotopes recently discovered make necessary an elastic relativistic view of such an "exact" science even as chemistry. One may look forward confidently to a further breaking down of the conceptual barriers of present-day categories of facts. This does not alter the fact that, as far as known, the heterogeneity of sets of natural phenomena must be admitted.

The qualities and the working principle of each heterogeneous category can be summarized in certain "laws" forming the basis for the study and exploration of such phenomena.

2. Among the various disciplines there can be shown to exist a certain hierarchial relation, the active principle of which is that the facts of the lower or simpler categories are pertinent to, but not explanatory for, those of the higher or more complex categories. Otherwise stated, the whole is greater than the sum of its parts. For example, the facts of chemistry and physics are pertinent to biology, but with perhaps rare exceptions offer inadequate explanation for

biological phenomena. The gap is filled only through a new *sort* of explanation.

Conversely, the essential principles peculiar to the higher or more complex categories have no meaning for the lower or more simple. Failure to observe faithfully the strictures imposed by these principles leads to the loose analogical thinking which dulls inquiry by its false appearance of explaining. Such absurdities as the "cellular soul" and reduction of human behavior to acid-base equilibrium are some natural consequences of such loose thinking.

Adolf Meyer sorts out the facts of science as shown in Figure 1.

Physics is concerned with mass (extension) and motion; chemistry with the properties of qualitatively discrete substances and the laws of their interaction. Beyond the physical and chemical data looms the biological, in which individuation first appears, in the

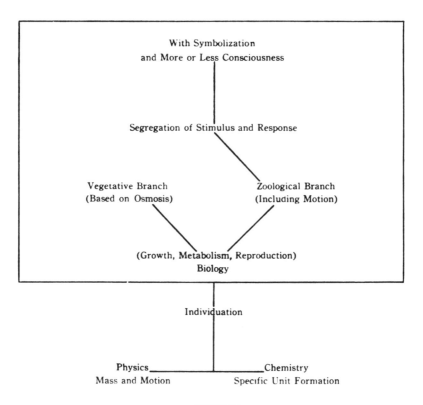

FIGURE 1.

sense of formation of individuals, including the chemical and physical data, but with important new properties, turning on growth,
development, metabolism, and reproduction. Within the biological
field are the subdivisions of (a) botany, in which the differentiating
facts are concerned with osmosis, and a fixed position relative to the
environment (except in the wide but chance distribution of the ger-
minal stages); and of (b) zoology, distinguished by motility, sensibility, and their organization into reflexes, simple delayed or con-
ditional reflexes (commonly called "learning"), and increased
adaptability to environmental conditions. Man emerges as a special
and a higher biological product, including within him all the data of
physics and chemistry and zoology, but distinguished by the greater
development of delayed reflexes as adaptive reactions, by the vast
development and use of symbols, especially those of language, and
by the hanging together of all these sensory, motor, and associative
performances in a special manner called "conscious."

In such a system the old contrast of mental and physical with its
prejudicial barriers and insolubilia is replaced by consideration of
degrees or levels of integration: Are the facts understood as nonmental, that is, as the qualities and activities of essentially detachable parts, organs, or systems (as treated in anatomy and physiology), or are they only intelligible in terms of mentally integrated
performances—of a sort indissolubly a function, overt or implicit,
of the total organism and having *meaning* as adaptive reactions in a
total situation?

Psychobiology then is the study of those functions distinctively
human, the things man is best known for, the mentally integrated
performances. The study demands knowledge of the physical sciences and of anatomy and physiology, but these in no wise explain
the phenomena under observation. Their explanation must be in
terms appropriate to the complexity of their level of integration: biological, but of a type operating with more or less consciousness, a
hanging together in a flow with symbolization.

A further inquiry has to do with the effects on total behavior of
variations, spontaneous or experimentally induced, in the nonmental
part-functions, and of the personal participation in mentally integrated performance. This constitutes a restatement of the unnecessary enigma of mind-body which has caused so much trouble for
centuries, and whose earlier solution ended in dualism, psychophysical parallelism, absolute materialism or absolute idealism, all of
which led to more polemical and prejudiced effort than constructive

and cooperative interest in finding the common ground and the allocation of legitimate fields of work.

The mentally integrated activities all have in common their essential quality of *meaning,* or *sense* and *direction,* which becomes clear when viewed in the light of the personal biographical record. Sensory stimulation may lead to reflex (nonmental) motor reactions, or they may, through experience, i.e., through temporal association including memory and anticipation, acquire symbolic meaning value and so play a part in complex mentally integrated functioning, in which the simple reflex response plays a subordinate role or may drop out entirely. The development of the mentally integrative functioning is not a matter of chance. It results in a more or less understandable way from the following factors:

(a) *The innate equipment,* (b) *the capacity for growth and organization,* and (c) *the modifying influences of immediate and more remote environment* on:

1. The sensory-motor equipment.
2. The instincts.
3. The emotions.
4. The conative tendencies.
5. The cognitive and associational assets, of memory, anticipation, discrimination, attention, etc.

Together they constitute the person-function or psychobiology— mentally integrated function in the service of life, or "ergasia" (A. Meyer)—mentally integrated person-function or behavior, implicit and overt.

All such function is organismal and in that sense "physical," but definitely more or less meaningfully connected, more or less conscious, i.e., integrated with the help of what the individual experiences with the help of symbolization, with mentation rather than any static "mind."

DIFFICULTIES ENCOUNTERED IN THE TEACHING OF PSYCHOBIOLOGY

The student is apt to say, "What difference does it make what philosophical view is held? How can that affect scientific pursuit?" It may be stated at the outset that the philosophies of science have resulted not from armchair speculation but from a practical demand for consistency and orderliness among the known facts. They result from the same processes by which the simplest and most isolated scientific observation is made available for further use: dependable specification of the facts, dependable methods, concepts, terms, and formulation.

The conspiracy of silence which has confronted psychobiology in the end probably resulted from three sources:

1. Overevaluation of the "personal," an extension of the doctrine that a man's home is his castle. Personal liberty has been so dearly won, and even today has been shown to be so fragile, that invasion of it is understandably resented. On the other hand, it would appear axiomatic that personal liberty flourishes best not in a state of mutual isolation and ignorance, but through understanding of human needs. The only way to know this is to be willing to share experience in a scientific quest.
2. Theological doctrine in the past has insisted on man's being subjected to a study wholly different from that accorded other natural phenomena. The apparently unbridgeable gap became filled by a cornerstone of dogma, quite unnecessary to that bolstering and development of the personal and social welfare, theology's proper ends.
3. Science itself has been slow in demanding that man be a proper object of its scrutiny. Even when psychology finally withdrew from philosophy and established itself as an independent discipline, there was a careful side-stepping of the main principles which should have guided such a study in favor of intensive research into special restricted items of human activity.

One of the great obstacles to active interest among students in the study of psychobiology is the discovery that the subject matter is largely within themselves. This is novel and disconcerting. When the object of study is external, little regard need be paid to subjective attitudes, objectivity is more easily held (sometimes illusory!) and results can be estimated in "grades," with some relation to the competitive character of the pursuit. Not so in psychobiology. When spoon feeding as so often practiced in preparatory schools is suddenly replaced by self-searching and a demand for independent thinking, the change is apt to be difficult. Active or passive resistance to the work then exerts itself with all the well-known rationalizations:

"The material is not well presented, not lucid; the instruction is dull; the basic sciences anatomy, chemistry, physiology, demand all the time." It is a rare student who openly sees and is able to talk about his difficulties with the study in terms of the status praesens of his own philosophy, because only the rare student has taken stock of his own philosophy and feels under obligation to know it.

The material of psychobiology—the personal data—is apt to appear prosaic, and the effort to organize the data is apt to be met with the attitude of indifference expressed by, "Everyone knows that"; yet the humdrum and prosaic are so only in their universality, requiring little scrutiny beyond the merest glance to be proved relatively unknown and unexplained. Efforts to inject showmanship into the study by undue emphasis on the unusual, as hypnosis, yoga, psychoanalytic metapsychology, or choice bits from psychopathology, are quite unnecessary and to be diligently avoided.

Granted that some philosophy of science is useful, what practical differences does it make whether that philosophy be the modern representative of the Aristotelian or of the Cartesian system?

Let us look at the position of the physician who holds to the Cartesian view. While asserting that those things distinctively human cannot be a subject for scientific inquiry, does he actually in practice ignore those things? Most assuredly not. He will admit that medical practice is part science, part "art," and, depending on his own personality make-up, he will be proud of his art or apologetic for its necessity. What goes by the name "art" is nothing but the intuitive recognition and use of those personal factors in oneself and others which a more rational view openly studies, organizes, and trains.

Dualism makes for a lack of frankness between physician and patient, for a need to soft-pedal any mention of "mental," for the introduction to the patient of the psychiatrist as a "neurologist," for a host of face-saving neurologizing and physiologizing explanations of human behavior, and for research programs whose aim is to put psychology on its feet by application of the "fundamental" sciences and thereby rob it of its only reason for existence.

Psychophysical parallelism is in no better position to offer satisfactory solutions to the material. Very soon devious explanation begins to run counter to universal common sense. And both absolute idealism and absolute materialism fail at the outset.

Let this be clear: The only study of man which offers unlimited opportunity is that which sees man in the general framework of biography with its biology and general science, which sees discrete units, wholes, and parts bound by the laws of integration.

FUNDAMENTAL CONCEPTIONS OF PSYCHOBIOLOGY

Such a view starting frankly with a biography acknowledges the age-old precept of the medical profession that our responsibility is to persons as well as to diseases; that the person is not merely the sum of the anatomical and physiological data of the component organs and systems, but is an integrate, not fully understandable or predictable from the anatomical and physiological data of the parts as such. It is the "he" or "she," living and in action, doing, feeling, thinking, remembering, anticipating—in short, creating a life record or biography. For many facts important for the understanding of a patient, we must look into his biographic record as a unitary individual, as an essential addition to the medical history of his cardiovascular, gastrointestinal, nervous, and other component systems.

This unitary activity of the individual, or "behavior," constitutes the material of psychobiology or ergasiology (from the Greek "ergasia" for "work, labor," introduced by Adolf Meyer because "behavior" has no plural or satisfactory adjective and is apt to exclude the mentation or subjective symbolization). In includes (1) overt behavior—the effective performances, as openly observable and intelligible as a talking picture is—and (2) implicit behavior—the more specifically ("centrally active and integrative") mental functions of sensations, perceptions, memories, fancies, etc., not as directly visible but open to inquiry and test. In practice overt and implicit behavior cannot be profitably separated. It is well to look upon overt behavior as full-fledged performance and the more "central" or implicit function as forerunner activity.

The anatomical and physiological basis for this unitary behavior has the brain as its principal integrating organ; without the forebrain hemispheres there can be only limited, if any, activity of this character. Nevertheless, behavior cannot be adequately described in neurological terms, as reflexes, synergias, tonus, etc., but only by what and how the person acts, feels, thinks, fancies, remembers, anticipates, and rendered in critical common-sense statements.

Theoretically the personality functions of the individual and group operate with meaning functions in varying degrees of consciousness or awareness. When physiological processes become long-circuited by means of delayed reflexes through the wealth of experience and associative material of the individual, they become amalgamated or brought into solution as a flow of personality functions with their sensations, perceptions, and memories. This transformation operates through the help of overt and economizing symbolization—attitudes, gestures, and expressions or thoughts bringing "meaning" or "sense" among the physiological processes. For example, weeping involves specific physiological activity of glands and muscles. When this specific physiological activity becomes long-circuited through the associative material and life experience of the individual, it emerges with sensations, perceptions, memories, anticipations, i.e., with meanings and differentiations, capable of influencing others and being observed and understood. Psychobiological functions therefore are not merely "mental" in the older sense of the data of introspection, but mentally integrated performances (or ergasias) of the individual, open to observation and interpretation, and playing their role in a sense of balance, disturbance and interpretation, or solution and ease.

Psychobiological functions deal with a number of items: (1) native assets, in (a) instinctual drives or performances, (b) the fundamental organismal rhythms of waking and sleeping, and variations in fitness and efficiency, and (c) intellectual differentiations or endowment; (2) acquired skills; (3) basic mood and its variations; (4) habits; (5) memories; (6) ambitions and vision of opportunities and anticipations; (7) imagination and fancy; and (8) reasoning. These are variously organized into an individual constitution, or organization of basic tendencies. The more or less stable and dependable constitutional structure is modified through growth and by the more plastic situational, life experience factors. In such a way the individual's life record unfolds. It may be sampled at any time for purposes of cross-section examination, giving a momentary symptomatological picture, completely understandable only in connection with the dynamics of the time-bound longitudinal view.

Since the psychobiological data have a basically history-making importance, it is no wonder that their study and understanding have long been the exclusive province of the spiritual guide, philosopher, sociologist, and educator. Traditional interest has been confined more to an abstract detachable "mind" or "soul" and little concerned with the organismal nature of that with which medicine has always worked. Medical men, dealing with both personality functions and the workings of organ systems, have a unique opportunity to observe human behavior, living out the events of a biography with their personal and social implications. When this biography is attended with a degree of orderly operation and satisfaction from life, it is called "normal." The conception of the normal comes from the knowledge of the self and the common-sense observation of others, and of hereditary and racial influences, social conditions, the variations of age from the developing infant to the declining aged—not merely by introspection, but always with a clear sense of objectivity.

AIMS OF PSYCHOBIOLOGY

Psychobiology has as ends therefore acquainting the student with (1) the sense of the importance of the meanings in activity, unfolding as a personal biography. In this, the purpose is not unlike that of the historian and dramatist; (2) personality organization at any given moment in cross section, the "subject organization"; (3) the range and variation of the normal.

The personal record of the subject is divided into the significant age periods for special study: Infancy, childhood, adolescence, maturity, involution. Some items of interest are:

Infancy (speechlessness)—up to the second year:

1. Details of maternal health during gestation, and birth data—duration, anesthesia, breathing, crying.
2. The physical status, with the health record.
3. Feeding, sleeping, bowel control—ease of establishment of habits.
4. The motility, for coordination, handedness, and skill.
5. Beginnings of language formation and conversation.
6. Emotional pattern: submissiveness, aggressiveness, dependence, "spoiled-child" tendencies, curiosity, detachment.
7. Personal interrelationships: playful cooperation; position in family, treatment by and of siblings; preference for parent.
8. Beginnings of visuomotor symbolizations and the utilization of space.
9. Sex data: spontaneous erections, their setting and apparent emotional factors related with. Curiosity—self-examination.
10. Concept formation and ingenuity in solving problems.

Childhood—2 years to puberty (10-15):

1. Development of language and motor skills.
2. Growth of social relations and adaptability.
3. Range and use of interests.

4. The school data.
5. The emotional pattern.
6. The family setting—attitude to siblings and to parents.
7. The sex data—curiosity, how satisfied.
8. Concept of the body configuration and of the ego.

Adolescence—the period of sexual maturation, period of rapid growth:

1. The sexual data—puppy love, awakening of the tender emotions. Menstruation and emissions—the preparedness for and reaction to. Beginning of growth of concept of family formation in a personal sense. Secondary sexual characteristics.
2. Social development: degree of active or passive participation.
3. Need for feeling of self-control—emancipation problems.
4. Personal attitude to religious considerations.
5. Ambitions.
6. Development of concept formation in direction of the more abstract.
7. The problem of surmounting apparently insurmountable contradictions such as selfishness and altruism, interest and boredom.

Maturity—from adolescence to the involution:

1. Fusion of the conative, cognitive, emotional and sexual assets into consistent drives for the personal and social good.
2. Relatively predictable behavior, subject to environmental stress, and to endogenous (constitutional and hereditary) liabilities, with a prevailing sense for responsibility of the performance.
3. Rather stable habits: eating, bowel control, sleep, work, play, use of leisure, and balance in required and spontaneous performance.

Involution—late and postclimacteric maturity and senescence:

1. Decreased work efficiency.
2. Health troubles—frailty.
3. Personality mellowing or change, with less aggression, substitution of indecisive consideration of issues for prompt action thereon.

4. Outcropping of early emotional and other personality attitudes previously during mature life kept under control.
5. Narrowing of field of interests, and lack of curiosity concerning new ones.
6. Return to the past.
7. Decline in intellectual assets.
8. Emotional lability.
9. Menopause and sexual (hormonal) decline, even or uneven, with comparable or paradoxical changes in psychosexual life.
10. Reduced nutritional and sleep demands.

COMPARISON WITH SOME OTHER METHODS
OF PERSONALITY STUDY

The personality study as described rests on the broad principles of psychobiological integration and should give a factual account of concrete performances. Starting with no axes to grind, and with a devotion to no special functions as the "core" of personality, the study reveals the person in action and the reasons for the action, as far as the objective evidence will allow. The study method keeps clear from systems of thought the result of clinical experiences with abnormal states, without, however, side-stepping issues pertinent for general personality study raised by those experiences. It relies on the historical method in the same way the dramatist or biographer does.

There are other methods of personality study, which may be used in conjunction with the study here outlined or independently. Since most of them rest on and are derivations from clinical findings, the reader is referred elsewhere for their details.

These methods are:

1. Introspective psychology, which holds that man is known only by the "inner" experience. Extreme views see the inner experience as the only "reality."

2. Graphology—in which certain personality traits are said to be revealed in the handwriting.

3. The form-color test of Rorschach—in which the subject's spontaneous perception of, and associations to, a sequence of ten ink blots, as concern for wholes, or details, form, color, or movement, of common or unusual content, with a wealth or scarcity of answers have been correlated empirically and logically with certain per-

sonality traits: the intelligence, the quality of the imagination, the mood, social adaptability, etc. (see 4 below).

4. The extravert-introvert concepts, as developed by Jung, and the "cyclothymic-schizothymic" concepts of Kretschmer, and the various "standardized tests" for their determination.

Jung popularized a dichotomy of personality into those with interests directed outward and those with the interests directed to the self.

Kretschmer approached the problem of the normal personality variants from his clinical observations of the relations between mental illness and body build. (See later chapters on psychiatric diagnosis.) By extension of these findings to the normal he defined two opposite types of personality, the cyclothymic with the pyknic body build (short, heavy, round chested), and the schizothymic, with the asthenic body build (tall, thin, flat chested).

The cyclothymic persons include the "talkative, cheerful; good humored; quiet, moody; complacent, pleasure-loving; active, practical."

The schizothymic include the "dignified, sensitive; unworldly, idealistic; calm, masterful; egoists and dull."

There are some correlations to be made with Rorschach test results. The cyclothymics react more to color, give emotionally tinged content, with practical ordinary concrete details; the schizothymics are more influenced by form, give unusual content with much movement, rich in imagination, and in abstraction, and less concerned with practical details.

5. The masculine-feminine dichotomy, and the determination of their personality traits by "standardized tests." Terman and Miles have recently studied masculinity and femininity by means of a questionnaire, the answers to which were assumed to be related to the basic issue of sexuality in its various expressions. The indecisive findings favor the conclusion that the fundamental assumptions of masculinity and femininity have little concreteness, or else the questions were poorly designed to elicit the data.

6. The conscious-unconscious polarizations as developed by the Freudian psychoanalytic school.

Psychoanalysis was developed by Freud and extended by his followers, at first as a technical method for treatment of certain sorts of mental disorders, but in later years it has offered a systematic account of personality formation and structure.

The basic concepts have to do with:

(a) The "unconscious," as the great reservoir of early established wishes, desires, drives of a sort not permitted expression by the personal and social ideal and forced from the conscious state into the unconscious by the act of "repression." Specifically, the *incest wish* declared to be present in all young children becomes so repressed.

(b) The personality is formed by balance between the two instincts—Eros, of the sexual, and the death instincts, representing essentially the life principle and the destructive tendencies, respectively. The fate of the sexual instinct or libido in its restricted meaning determines largely the quality of the personality structure and functioning, the principal types being dominantly in chronological order of appearance narcissistic, oral, anal, phallic, and genital in the development of the libido. Each stage of libidinous fixation determines a syndrome of personality traits: narcissistic (after Narcissus, the self-admirer of Greek mythology), denoting the self-lover, the ingrowing, egocentric, introversive (Jung), with a preponderance of wishful fancy unchecked by reality; oral, with the libidinous impulses centered on the lips and mouth, and with the presence of sucking, mouthing, chewing, etc., as evidences of the continuance of pleasure-giving propensities of the area; anal—interest in the rectum and anus, the excreta, with over-cleanliness, meticulousness, obsessive trends, penuriousness, and a tendency to place blame elsewhere for personal failure; phallic, related to fixation on the aggressive organ and to homosexual tendencies; genital, the normal mature adult with adequate intersexual capacity.

In normal development each stage is a sequel to the preceding one, but residues of previous stages are to be found throughout later ones.

(c) The facts of the unconscious—the repressed material, and especially the data of infantile and childhood sexual levels of development—are brought to light only through the circumvention of the conscious waking self, which is continually on guard as the censor to prevent their emergence. This circumvention is accomplished by means of "free association" under the condition of "transference," by the interpretation of dreams in their latent content, by slips of the tongue, i.e., in all those activities in which conscious awareness may be presumed to be lacking. Since the waking state is devoted to overcoming primitive impulses and desires, it follows that the unconscious wishes are more or less the opposite of those actually consciously displayed, e.g., one loves because he desires to deny his real hates, or because the loved one resembles someone for whom love is forbidden, etc. The conscious is represented as playing a very subordinate role in actual human performance, with the proper goal of life being the increase in this factor at the expense of the unconscious.

The strong sense of motivation from universal childhood experience in all behavior is apparent from this.

Freud sees the personality structure as finally constituted divided into three provinces with unlike functions:

1. The id, entirely unconscious, harboring the crude instincts seeking expression.
2. The ego, split off from the id by contact with reality through the sensory-motor apparatus, whose function is to maintain harmony between the id and external reality. It is largely conscious.
3. The superego, largely conscious, the repressing agency, whose function is to keep the id under cover. It arises as a residue of the Oedipus situation, when the incest wish is repressed through the disapproval of the parent of the same sex. The incorporation of the parental repressing tendency into the self (by "introjection") is the beginning of the superego.

The ego is under obligation to the id to find suitable ways of expression, to reality of the external world, and to the superego as conscience.

7. The variants of the psychoanalytic school, the individual psychology of Adler, stressing the roles of aggression and submission and of organ inferiority and its compensation in a will to power; and Jung's analytical psychology, stressing the racial and cultural, as well as the personal, "unconscious."

Adler and Jung were early disciples of Freud, but broke with the master on the question of the all-importance of the sexual principle. Adler saw the practical issue of desire for power and reward as motivating all human performance, often enough in an attempt to overcome original constitutional inferiority.

Jung became interested in the broad cultural and racial deep motivations in addition to the more personal ones. The treatment of human motivations is at once more broadly based than Freud's, but also somewhat mystical.

Both Adler and Jung rely largely on the method of free association, dream analysis, etc., for the material of the personality structure and functioning.

8. Behaviorism of Watson, in which human behavior is reduced to certain primitive adaptive reactions and their elaboration through environmental influences in a thoroughgoing mechanistic fashion. Watson no doubt was influenced by distrust of the introspectionism of the time and attracted to the schematic simplifications of the Pavlovian school. As with the latter (see 9), the explanations of human behavior offered by this school are remarkable for their mechanistic conception, their ruthless simplicity and the illusion that new words offer a surer understanding than the simple facts in old garb.

9. Conditioned reflexes of Pavlov, resting on animal experimentation, applied by analogy to the human and reducing behavior to the simple neurophysiological terms of "excitation" and "inhibition."

10. Gestalt psychology, which recognizes the principle that the human performance cannot be explained adequately as the summation of the part performances, but that things occur in wholes of integrates. It has been applied most extensively to the field of sensory perception. It proceeds to the effort of clarification of behavior by experiment with a reduction to quasi-mathematical rules, with "tension," "fields," "vectors," and has been less concerned with the historical data.

Introspective psychology was obviously a one-sided performance, and eventually ran into the difficulty of explaining why the human perceives as he does, so paving the way for historically-minded and for Gestalt psychologies.

Gestalt psychology, conditioned reflexes, and behaviorism draw their strength largely from the appeal to the "exact" methods of the laboratory, and conditioned reflexes and behaviorism also from the analogy with neurophysiology with its relatively simple formulations. Developed as reactions to mystical elements in the older introspective psychology, which saw in the inner experience the only reality, these methods have added illuminating data concerning fragments of behavior, and the neurophysiological participations.

The various analytic methods are the outcome of the use of special methods, concepts, and attitudes, designed to record the doings of a hidden force which makes man behave as he does. The vitalism so conceived has resulted in an enormous amount of work, which, however, leaves one uncertain how much is naively factual, how much the result of the methods, how much interpretation elevated to the status of belief. These methods have certainly cast illumination on the less obvious features of personality, and in so doing have created new test situations themselves needing further clarification.

The difficulty of all these methods in producing a rounded picture of the person in action derives from the following, singly or in combination:

1. Blindness to the plain facts of integration in favor of the outmoded mind-body dualism, or of absolute materialism.
2. The assumption of certain limited items as the "core" of personality—e.g., the sexual instinct, simple reflexes, natural Gestalten, the modern equivalents of the mystical soul which these systems fought to dethrone.
3. The reduction of human behavior to descriptive adjectives on the basis of laboratory tests, presuming to derive from the cross-section performance a finality of description legitimately made only with due regard for the historical-longitudinal data.
4. The errors inherent in any transfer of behavioristic data from laboratory animals to man.
5. The false assumption that better understanding of behavior is achieved by giving to performance *names* likely to carry in the context meaning not inherent in the performance itself. The names used are largely analogues of terms used in the physical sciences or borrowings from mythology.
6. Oversystematization of the material through exclusion of data not fitting into the scheme, with the appeal to half truth, and making belief in the system paramount.

The leading features of unprejudicial genetic-dynamic psychobiology rest on:

1. The partly historical, partly experiment-like formulation of the events and facts as found.
2. The open operative type of definition.
3. The reduction to a generally applicable concept of fact and the principle of concrete quasi-experimental inquiry. Concreteness versus mere analogy.
4. The willingness to recognize patterns figuring as anticipation and purpose.
5. Willingness to include standards of effort and responsibility.

6. Avoidance of mere either-or dichotomy in favor of frank reciprocities and multiple interrelations and necessity of intelligent selection of leading items in a pluralism with consistency.

REFERENCES

1. Meyer, A. Conditions for a Home of Psychology in the Medical Curriculum, *J. Abnorm. Psychol., 7*: 313, 1912-13.
2. Dandy, W. E. Changes in Our Conceptions of Localization of Certain Functions of the Brain, *Am. J. Physiol., 93*: No. 2, June, 1930.
3. Stanley, W. M. Tobacco Mosaic Virus in Crystalline Form From Tobacco Plants, *Science, 81*: 644, 1935.

Historical

Meyer, A. Objective Psychology or Psychobiology With Subordination of the Medically Useless Contrast of Mental and Physical, *J. A. M. A., 65*: 860, 1915.
Idem. The Justification of Psychobiology as a Topic of the Medical Curriculum, *Psychol. Bull., 12*: 328, 1915.
Idem. Scope and Teaching of Psychobiology, *J. A. Am. M. Col., 10*: 93, 1935.
Idem. Psychobiology in the First Year of Medical School, *J. A. Am. M. Col., 10*: 365, 1935.
Idem. Misconceptions at the Bottom of "Hopelessness of All Psychology," *Psychol. Bull., 4*: 170, 1907.
Idem. The Contribution of Psychiatry to the Understanding of Life Problems. In *A Psychiatric Milestone,* Bloomingdale Hospital Centenary, 1821-1921, New York, 1921, pp. 21-54.
Stanley, W. M. & Loring, H. S. Tobacco Mosaic Virus in Crystalline Form From Tomato Plants, *Science, 83*: 85, 1936.
Singer, C. *A Short History of Biology. A General Introduction to the Study of Living Things,* Oxford, 1931, pp. 37-39.
Müller-Freienfels, R. *The Evolution of Modern Psychology.* Translated by Béran Wolfe, MD, New Haven, 1935, Yale University Press.
Adler, M. *What Man Has Made of Man,* Chapter 2. New York, 1937, Longmans Green & Co.

General

Müller-Freienfels, R. *The Evolution of Modern Psychology.* New Haven, 1935, Yale University Press.
Woodworth, R. S. *Contemporary Schools of Psychology.* New York, 1931, The Ronald Press Co.

Graphology

Diethelm, O. The Personality Concept in Relation to Graphology and Rorschach Test. In the *Biology of the Individual,* the Proceedings of the Association for Research in Nervous and Mental Disease, *14*: 278, 1934.

Rorschach

Rorschach, H. *Psychodiagnostik,* ed. 2, Bern and Berlin, 1932, Hans Huber.

Masculinity, Femininity

Terman, L. M. & Miles, C. C. *Sex and Personality: Studies in Masculinity and Femininity.* New York, 1936.

Psychoanalysis

Freud, S. *New Introductory Lectures on Psychoanalysis.* London, 1933, Hogarth Press.

Behaviorism

Watson, J. B. *Behaviorism.* The People's Institute Publishing Co., New York, 1925.

Conditioned Reflexes

Pavlov, I. P. *Lectures on Conditioned Reflexes*—Translated by W. H. Gantt, MD, New York, 1928, International Publishers.

Eleanor Clarke Slagle:
Founder and Leader
in Occupational Therapy

Karen Diasio Serrett

Although Eleanor Clark Slagle is well known as a founder of occupational therapy in this country, few of her written works have been readily available to occupational therapists. She is primarily known clinically for her work with psychiatric patients, and especially for setting up programs of habit training in many hospitals. Slagle and Meyer worked together for many years, and elsewhere in this volume is Meyer's tribute to Slagle. It seems fitting that the following excerpts from her writings be included in this volume.

AIMS OF PROGRAMS

Slagle, in describing her work in the New York State hospitals, described the following aims in her work:

> To know the individual problems of each hospital, to seek cooperation and to cooperate to the fullest possible extent in the effort to motivate as many as possible of the large number of patients living in the so-called 'back wards'; to establish habit training classes where none existed; to help in grading the established occupational efforts; and to help in stimulating among hospital employees a sense of the larger opportunity to help patients to readjust themselves, both socially and industrially, through organized occupation. (Slagle, 1924, p. 98)

> In the light of our present understanding of psychiatry and methods of prophylaxis we are bound to assume that one of the great needs presented by our state hospitals today will have passed forever within the next ten years. In that time we should

101

have eliminated the so-called back wards. No matter how highly trained occupational workers may be in class, it takes consecration and a genuine love of the human family to undertake the direction of and participation in habit training classes among patients who have been in hospitals anywhere from five to twenty years and who have steadily gone down almost to the lower animal level. To arrange a twenty-four hour schedule for these patients, a schedule in which physicians, nurses, attendants, and occupational therapeutists play a part has not been an easy matter. But we knew that we could not train workers for selected groups, unless we included work for that great group that had landed in the discard of life—they were entitled to a chance—and the writer of this paper cannot pay too high a tribute to all who have helped create such a program or to the pupils who have been willing to participate in it. Their work has demonstrated what re-education really means for mental patients and every once in a while the discard has yielded a patient fully reclaimed for home and community activity. (Slagle, 1922, p. 13)

ON TEACHING HABIT TRAINING

"So our first duty in training the occupational worker for mental patients is to show them what the problem is; that, for the most part, our lives are made up of habit reactions. Occupation used remedially serves to overcome some habits, to modify others and construct new ones, to the end that habit reaction will be favorable to the restoration and maintenance of health. It is important that the pupils should understand the interdependence of the mental and physical and to also realize that a mental handicap is greater than a physical disability, because of the traditional prejudice against a person who has suffered from mental disease. *In habit training, we show clearly an academic psychology factor that the occupational worker must always bear in mind with mental patients—that is, the necessity of requiring attention, of building on the habit of attention—attention thus becomes application, voluntary and in time agreeable"* (emphasis added).

"The necessity of never ending activity along this line with the reception service, and with the large, unemployed, deteriorating groups found in every state institution, can not be too strongly emphasized.

"Habit building for dementia praecox is highly important. If the disorganization of habit is basic with this type, then we must more and more concern ourselves with elaborations on the work already begun in many hospitals.

". . . From habit training we advance to the kindergarten group. Our prospective teachers must be taught kindergarten methods as applied to a re-educational program. We must show the ways and means of stimulating the special senses. The employment of color, music, simple exercises, games, and story telling along with occupations, the gentle ways and means we use in educating a child, are equally important in re-educating the adult.

". . . From kindergarten through grades in which all manual exercises are graded to meet the needs of the individual patient, patients are advanced through these grades in which a certain underlying pedagogical principle is observed in the application of occupational therapy. That is, grading from the simple to the complex, passing from the known to the unknown, the tasks must be of increasing interest and requiring an increasing degree of concentration.

". . . Progressing to the occupational center or 'curative workshop,' as it is frequently called, the pupil observes the patient in his evolutionary process and is gratified at last to use her full craft knowledge gained in her technical studies and to see really beautiful work accomplished by the individual.

"From the occupational center with its busy round of splendid activity, the student reviews and sees, as it were, the picture of his imaginary world, the desirability of substituting varying interests, the inhibitions, the whole emotional field and the relation of all the steps taken in helping to create a suitable balanced program of work, rest, play for mental patients.

"The occupational center serves more or less as a proving ground for the adaptation of the patient to an entirely new environment and to other members of the group who have been advanced to this point for various specialized observation. From this center patients are frequently paroled, others are carefully graded and assigned to the pre-industrial group. The student has by this time learned the system of occupational analysis and begins to see why such a system is of enormous value and also begins to understand our terminology. The work on the wards or work in the pre-industrial group may contribute to vocational outlook.

". . . The success of any program of rehabilitation—important as all its stages are and the promptness with which it is accomplished—depend to a very large measure upon occupational therapy, the persistency, versatility, and patience of the occupational therapeutist." (Slagle, 1922, 14-17)

Later, Slagle and Robeson elaborated further on their view of habit:

"Because habits are formed in all spheres of activity—mental, physical, and social—and because an attempt is made to make the life of the patient in an institution as normal as possible, no program of treatment would be complete without directed physical and recreational activities. These hold an important place in our occupational program. . . .

"Dr. Salmon has said . . . 'Progressive daily achievement is the only way manhood and self-respect can be regained.'

"The easiest habit to form is that of following the line of least resistance. This applies to the teacher as well as patient and the rehabilitation of the patient can only be achieved by a definite development and reorganization of mental processes by means of a constructive and progressive method of treatment. Any occupation given for a curative purpose ceases to be treatment when it becomes mechanical." (Slagle and Robeson, 1931, 30-31)

It is clear that Slagle built on the thinking of William James; he is quoted in her training Syllabus:

" 'The moment one tries to define what habit is, one is led to the fundamental properties of matter . . . Habit diminishes the conscious attention with which our acts are performed.' (William James)

"Habit training is the first step in the State program of occupational therapy. It has two purposes:

1. The reclamation and rehabilitation of the patient: (a) to return the patient to the community if possible, or (b) to make him a more acceptable member of the hospital community.
2. Resulting economic advantages: (a) the patient becomes less destructive and untidy. The savings on clothes destroyed and laundry. (b) requires less care and supervision.

"What is meant by habit training? Applied to our hospital patients it means re-education in decent habits of living. Re-education follows the same growth and development as normal education. Broadly speaking, 'Re-education is substituting better habits (for bad habits) or the building of new habits to replace those which have been lost.' There is no *general* habit, no *general* memory, that is common to all mankind. It is *individual* habit and memory. Every one builds his or her own. *'Habit psychology' is the only basis on which to re-educate* [emphasis added]. Ideals are a *continued* attitude of mind (habit). Skill is a habit of performance. . . . Adolf Meyer describes dementia praecox as 'disorganized habits.' . . . Kraepelin says of dementia praecox 'What is necessary for them is occupation which alone can preserve, by exercise, the capabilities which still remain to them and prevent them from wholly sinking into dullness.' '' (Slagle and Robeson, 1931, 30-35)

PERSPECTIVES ON HISTORY
OF OCCUPATIONAL THERAPY

Slagle also taught from a series of 15 principles set forth by the American Occupational Therapy Association. The syllabus for training developed by Slagle and Robeson included a brief history of occupational therapy:

"This training course was, without any question, the outgrowth of a strong interest not only in mental hygiene as a movement, but in the care of mental patients, particularly wards of the state. This was brought about by the publication of ''A Mind That Found Itself,'' by Clifford Whittingham Beers. Through the interest aroused by the publication of this book and the challenge contained in this remarkable human document regarding the care and treatment of those suffering from mental diseases, the first course of training in occupations for the mentally sick was established in the Chicago school.

"It was natural that Illinois, with its outstanding group of humanitarian workers at this period, should be among the first to evolve the idea of a course of special instruction for workers in state hospitals. Among the group mentioned as sponsoring these first classes in occupational measures were Julia Lathrop, then member of the State Board of Control and afterwards head of the Children's Bureau in Washington; Jane Addams, of Hull House; Dr. Adolf Meyer, of Johns Hopkins Hospital; Edward Worst, superintendent of manual training, Public Schools of Chicago, and others almost equally prominent.

". . . It will be recalled that, due to the interest of such men as Dr. William Welch of Johns Hopkins University; William James, of Harvard University; Dr. Adolf Meyer, Dr. Thomas W. Salmon, Dr. Lewellys Barker and others, and to Clifford Beer, the National Committee for Mental Hygiene was established. . . .

"With such an impetus in the beginning, it is little wonder that the work has advanced, particularly where those inspired by this group have taken up further study and practice of treatment by occu pation." (Slagle and Robeson, 1931, 12-13)

Slagle and Robeson also commented about occupational therapy.

"Note the broadness of this field—'any activity, mental or physical.' This would cover ploughing a field or studying a foreign language, handicrafts, physical exercises, baseball, etc., just so long as these activities were regularly prescribed and guided for their therapeutic value to the patient." (p. 17)

They stated the purpose of occupational therapy was

"To reconstruct, to rebuild or re-educate the patient, (a) mentally; (b) physically, and (c) socially according to the individual need and to the highest capability of the patient." (p. 19)

ORGANIZATIONAL AND PROGRAM DEVELOPMENT ASPECTS

Slagle is widely credited with introducing habit training in many states and countries. It is clear she had much organizational skill that was applied in these settings. These organizational skills can be seen in her description of occupational therapy program development in New York State:

"Our first step was toward a unified program of occupational therapy; but one which would, at the same time, allow of wide individual freedom to the superintendents of the various hospitals. In other words, we felt that our duty to the work called for an attitude of advisory helpfulness towards those directly responsible for the care and treatment of the patients, rather than an attitude of 'direction.'

"The last thing we had in mind was an immediate or later

upheaval of all the consistent and good work already established in the state hospitals. It seemed reasonable, however, in view of the good results obtained by a coordinated, state-wide system in other states, to feel that in New York we should not be satisfied with mediocre results when, by systematic effort and intensive study, a comprehensive program could be worked out.

"Obviously, the first practical measure to be undertaken was a study of the existing work in each hospital, but from the beginning the studies were constructive and the ready cooperation of the superintendents and of all concerned made it possible to undertake developmental work in many hospitals almost simultaneously with the preliminary study of the particular institution. . . .

". . . The response to the effort to put such a program into operation will always stand out as one of the most inspiring experiences of our professional career. On every hand within the hospitals there has been such a cordial spirit of invitation to lead the way, and it is due to this fine spirit that a rare record of accomplishment has been made possible. Success in work of this nature never depends upon one person alone; therefore it is not only just, but a pleasure, to pay tribute to those who have helped to bring the ultimate program of the commission nearer realization; namely, the personnel of the hospitals, from the superintendents downwards, whose cordial cooperation and ready help have made pleasant the work of a very strenuous year." (Slagle, 1924, p. 98)

"It has been my privilege to organize work in different states. Of course, you have different circumstances in each state. I went to Michigan to help start a training school for nurses in connection with the state hospital. It was considered almost impossible. There were strikes, there were various internal uprisings, and they were very difficult to overcome, and the work was considered very successful there." (Slagle, 1914, p. 27)

Slagle, seemingly for reasons of practicality, stressed the importance of a physician prescription:

> "I tried to make a point,—that no one should ever be admitted to the classes who is not sent by a physician. The classes are not carried on to get rid of some patients who sit about the wards in an apathetic condition. That is the only one point that I over-emphasize. . . ." [Dr. Klopp, in response] "I fully agree with that statement. Furthermore, that the industrial in-

structor shall be informed as to the particular mental characteristics of that patient, so that she may better understand, and
possibly assist in the occupying of that patient from a therapeutic standpoint.'' [Slagle, in response]: ''I think that relieves the
director of the scientific responsibility that might be considered his or her responsibility. That has come up several times
in my work. What scientific background have you for putting
that patient in occupational work, and of course, I very quickly
respond by saying 'That is not my affair. That is for the scientific men on the staff to answer.' '' (Slagle, 1914, p. 28)

Slagle's later writings do not refer to any viewpoint that differs
from the one mentioned above, but her answer makes clear she was
adroit at maneuvering in the culture and organizational climate of
her times. Not only was she knowledgeable about the basic premises
of functionalism and pragmatism, she was also very skilled at taking
William James' fundamental statement about habit (published elsewhere in this volume) and operationalizing it widely and with
creditable results.

REFERENCES

Slagle, E.C. (1924) A year's development of occupational therapy in New York State Hospi-
tals. *Modern Hosp.*, *22*:1: 98-104.
Slagle, E.C. (1922) Training aides for mental patients. *Arch. Occup. Ther.*, *1*:1: 11-17.
Slagle, E.C. (1934) Occupational Therapy: Recent methods and advances in the United
States. *Occup. Ther. and Rehab.*, *13*:5: 289-298.
Slagle, E.C. (1937) Editorial: From the heart. *Occup. Ther. and Rehab.*, *16*:5: 343-345.
Slagle, E.C. (1914) History of the development of occupation for the insane. *Maryland
Psychiat. Quart.*, *4*: 14-32.
Slagle, E.C. & Robeson, H.A. (1941) *Syllabus for Training of Nurses in Occupational Ther-
apy.* Utica, NY: State Hospital Press.
Slagle, E.C. (1938) Occupational therapy. *Trained Nurse and Hosp. Rev.*, *100*:4: 375-382.

Address in Honor
of Eleanor Clarke Slagle

Adolf Meyer

It is a great privilege to have an opportunity to speak on this occasion which honors a friend and long-time coworker, our Mrs. Eleanor Clarke Slagle, as a person and as the personification of occupational therapy. Presidents and officers have come and gone but for 20 years Mrs. Slagle has brought into the field just that kind of personality which proved highly fruitful and auspicious: she has been, not a dictator, not a boss, but a leader by example, a human being and human factor among human beings, a cultivator of human relationships, in gathering around herself coworkers and in making coworkers of the patients. Such is the human being Mrs. Slagle and what she means to us and to the thousands of patients who have been and are still reached by her and her pupils. And inseparable from this personal human side, there stands before us the nature and character of the product of her work and the spirit and philosophy her life and life-work exemplify, that which brings us together in this assembly and in this large and impressive organization.

This gathering and the work achieved by this body with Mrs. Slagle as the head worker are enough of a testimonial for a cause and its leading and stabilizing captain. Obviously Mrs. Slagle has had her ideal not only in perpetuating herself in a special role but in training a rank and file ever able to furnish timber for leadership from the ranks and in the ranks, and growth from the ranks.

For 20 years, from the beginning of our organization, Mrs. Slagle has, as treasurer and secretary, done that work of continuity which with changing presidents and changing topics represents the very constitution of this growing force in the ranks of dealing with those who, for a time and sometimes for good, are forced into that army that needs shelter and protection and among whom the work of

Delivered by Dr. Adolf Meyer at a testimonial banquet in honor of Eleanor Clarke Slagle at Atlantic City, September 14, 1937.

This moving tribute from Meyer to Slagle has, until now, remained unpublished and largely unknown.

restoring health and better ways of prevention and achievement of
the handicapped brings care and cure.

In these days in which we are perhaps too much inclined to look
upon leadership as a profession, and upon professional agitators as
the reapers of honor and power, it is a tremendous satisfaction to see
one of the chief workers completing 20 years in that office which
personifies the very constitution of this body. Mrs. Slagle and Dr.
Dunton have been the spirits in the ranks and from the ranks and for
the ranks, not imposed managers, but the souls of the essence of the
work, giving freely of their time and experience while carrying on
the work itself.

In the great division of labor we need continuity and examples
that survive the changes and are embodiments of the very essentials
which only the best workers can perpetuate in steady growth, in
stability of motion and promotion, those who see that ever new deals
are fair deals, deals embodying the wisdom of those who do and actually work and never cease to grow and to create.

Growth and work and achievement and attainment are all a function of that one virtual commodity time, that steady rhythm of day
and night, of seasons and years, not a mere eternal return but eternal
progression. No two days can be quite the same, and no two years;
but there has to be an element of continuity and cohesion; and for
this it takes those starting with enough personality, capable of maintaining themselves and of remaining forces and centers of growth.
And as in the nature of humanity, generation follows generation, the
young work beside the old and the old work beside the young, those
capable of being the bearers of continuity are few and rare and, we
are glad to see, honored and sought as the very essence of progress.

Mrs. Slagle comes from the same source and soil that gave me my
first opportunities and encouragement: the opportunity to realize the
need for more, the need for growth, the opportunity to find similarly
minded forces and the spirit of action that has to go with knowledge
and vision to make it both fertile and practical: Illinois, large needs
and large enterprises, a whole group of aspiring forces and engaging
problems, needs in practice and needs in hospitals, close to Mis-
souri, wanting to be shown and shown by actual work and performances. The educator, the social worker and the physician were
bound to get together. Miss Lathrop was one of the great links. As
the great gardener Froebel in education and his pupil Grossman in
the therapeutic training of psychopaths by work recognized the need
of a setting for work and for therapy in sound use of time, so there

was the shaping of an atmosphere of work and action at Kankakee, encouraged by the social spirit about Hull House, all working for the training by action and not only by word. The old ideal of the Middle Ages, pray and work, took real form in the union of one's best thought and work, and when we opened the Phipps Clinic for action, Miss Lathrop was able to lend us Mrs. Slagle as the model and instigator of workmanship in the service of therapy. That the greatest benefit for the sufferer was to come from the philosophy of time and its use and from the right person to exemplify it was natural in the pragmatic atmosphere of the middle west and Mrs. Slagle brought the fruit of experience to our new center. She started us and, like all good workers, inspired others, so that, when she was needed for more and more training of new forces, she left with us the workers who carried on while she was drawn into that field of training and teaching and organizing, that did so much in the emergencies of that international madness called war and again for the needs arising from the madness and the immaturity and blunderings even in peace. As a contributor to the philosophy of time and life, as a cultivator of life and health in activity, Mrs. Slagle has become a guide, philosopher and friend of hundreds and hundreds, and as I said, the embodiment of example and principle. What she has added in the nearly twenty-five years since she came to help us is a proud record, a rare fulfillment of a life still growing and still progressing.

The demands of actual life and work where it is most needed have wrought a wonderful change in turning psychology from esoteric contemplation into the service of actual life. Real needs and real opportunities have led us into modern psychobiology and a science of human nature and behavior. And the basis of this modern psychobiology is not mere analysis and preaching of license, but a study and cultivation of the person and action. This is how the old principle of engaging patients in activity has become the basic setting of all modern therapy. Pathology is no longer a kind of gloating over what can be found at autopsy. It is the study of the mistakes and maladjustments, the failures of man to use his best sense and opportunities. Mistakes become damage and damage becomes disease and disease in turn has to be brought back to where it is treated as "poor work" to be replaced by good and helpful work. This is the role of occupational therapy, not merely making a lot of stereotyped articles but releasing or implanting and fostering action with the reward and joy of achievement. I have heard Mrs. Slagle quote from a passage in the first paper I ever wrote on the treatment of

nervous and mental disorders, addressed to the Chicago Pathological Society in February, 1893, nearly forty-five years ago, in which
I asked my colleagues for the discussion of the kind of work which
could be expected from and recommended to American ladies. I do
not know why I picked on the ladies; I suppose because the doctors
present were all men and I felt I knew them. I said: 'Experience
alone can give suggestions in this line.' I called it mental hygiene,
foreshadowing what I now mean by "mind," the person in action,
good or bad, helpful and effective or mere restlessness, often over-
active only as the result of fatigue and mismanagement.

I should like to be able to voice adequately what so many of my
patients have gained through Mrs. Slagle and her pupils and what it
all means not only for the sufferer but also for the healthy of our
time. When the development of machinery supersedes the driving
power of necessity in the development of habits and possibilities of
work, we turn to the ingenuity of those who know the creative possibilities available not only for the sick but for the rank and file of
those with "time on their hands."

From reveling in thoughts of eternity, we now have the great task
to inject again the joys of activity of the day so that we may make a
return of the pleasure of the day's work an efficient competitor with
the mere pleasure and glamor of night life. We are grateful to Mrs.
Slagle and her pupils and coworkers for their devotion and skill and
creative zeal and achievements in the furtherance of the joy and
rewards of work and creation.

It must be a great satisfaction to Mrs. Slagle to see the onward
march of what had but slender beginnings. There is a need of leisure
for the spreading of the wisdom that has come from the wide experience under difficult conditions. As wisdom grows there comes
the demand for a spreading into wider usefulness. Today we have
come into a period of prostitution of the capacity and love for work
to the service of the something and the somebody else of mere
wages. We have more and more cause to search for the natural in-
ducements to work and the opportunities for new creative principles. We have to study work for its own rewards and to honor and
cherish it and to cultivate it so as to make it deserve the honor and
joy. Working under the difficulties met by the psychiatric occupational worker should and will give us much material for a usuable
knowledge of the relation of person and work, worker and work,
and worker and leadership.

What is the work one can love and live with and live on? What are the conditions of work that are needed if the worker is to love the work and to live on and through it?

I shall never forget the deplorable words of a Secretary of Labor in a discussion of immigration. He told us we needed some immigration to get labor to do the dirty work which no American parent would want his children to do.

We occupational workers know that there is no work that cannot be shaped so as to find its worker able to get satisfaction from the doing and the result.

In these days in which continuity of purpose seems overshadowed by doctrines of change and where leadership in a democratic sense threatens to be belittled and to degenerate in other lands into high-power dictatorships, it is a matter of great joy and cheer to see respect and honor brought to a leader of unusual modesty and gentleness.

In the midst of talk and reality of change we see careers of continuity of progress, of action and creativeness in the ranks, and as part of the ranks.

We see those natural and inspiring instances in which a rare individual becomes a live and effective example of ideas and ideals as the living and active person, and persons expressive of ideals.

And we are glad to see those persons who become living symbols of great movements and realizations, in the midst of the younger and the budding generations, sharing with them the experience of a lifetime and the spirit of everbudding youth.

It is the pride of democracy to cherish its leaders as parts of the ranks, as influence by example, and as recipients of recognition and of fellowship in the rank and file.

We like to see it brought home that a lifetime of work and service and devotion and leadership in a cause also finds its recognition, and recognition and esteem its expression.